Anti-Inflammatory Diet for Beginners: The Complete Guide to Healing Your Immune System, Restoring Health and Naturally Remedying Arthritis & Chronic Fatigue

By Jason Michaels

The book contains 2 manuscripts:

Anti-Inflammatory Diet: Make these simple, inexpensive changes to your diet and start feeling better within 24 hours!

Anti-Inflammatory Diet: The Complete Guide for Managing Rheumatoid Arthritis and Healing Chronic Disease Using Healthy Food

Table of Contents

Anti-Inflammatory Diet: The Complete Guide for Managing Rheumatoid Arthritis and Healing Chronic Disease Using Healthy Food

The following eBook is reproduced below with the goal of providing information that is as accurate and reliable as possible. Regardless, purchasing this eBook can be seen as consent to the fact that both the publisher and the author of this book are in no way experts on the topics discussed within and that any recommendations or suggestions that are made herein are for entertainment purposes only. Professionals should be consulted as needed prior to undertaking any of the action endorsed herein.

This declaration is deemed fair and valid by both the American Bar Association and the Committee of Publishers Association and is legally binding throughout the United States.

Furthermore, the transmission, duplication or reproduction of any of the following work including specific information will be considered an illegal act irrespective of if it is done electronically or in print. This extends to creating a secondary or tertiary copy of the work or a recorded copy and is only allowed with an expressed written consent from the Publisher. All additional right reserved.

The information in the following pages is broadly considered to be a truthful and accurate account of facts and as such any inattention, use or misuse of the information in question by the reader will render any resulting actions solely under their purview. There are no scenarios in which the publisher or the original author of this work can be in any fashion deemed liable for any hardship or damages that may befall them after undertaking information described herein.

Additionally, the information in the following pages is intended only for informational purposes and should thus be thought of as universal. As befitting its nature, it is presented without assurance regarding its prolonged validity or interim quality. Trademarks that are mentioned are done without

written consent and can in no way be considered an endorsement from the trademark holder.

Medical Disclaimer

This book is not intended as a substitute for the medical advice of physicians. The reader should regularly consult a physician in matters relating to his/her health and particularly with respect to any symptoms that may require diagnosis or medical attention.

Please consult your physician before starting any diet or exercise program.

Any recommendations given in this book are not a substitute for medical advice.

Anti-Inflammatory Diet

Make these simple, inexpensive changes to your diet and start feeling better within 24 hours!

By Jason Michaels

Introduction

Congratulations on downloading *Anti-Inflammatory Diet: Make these simple, inexpensive changes to your diet and start feeling better within 24 hours!* and thank you for doing so.

The following chapters will discuss how the anti-inflammatory diet isn't a diet in the traditional meaning of the term, because its intended purpose isn't weight loss, though people do often lose weight when following it. It's also not a diet you follow for a limited time until you reach your goal and then quit. Rather it's a true lifestyle change focused on anti-inflammatory principles with the purpose of providing stable energy, and adequate vitamins, essential fatty acids, minerals, fiber, and defensive anti-inflammatory phytonutrients to reach and maintain better health.

This book is written to help people understand aspects of inflammation and how the typical American diet contributes to it. It looks at the effects of the resulting chronic inflammation on health and how chronic low-grade inflammation can even contribute to weight gain and other health issues. Once equipped with this understanding, you'll learn what you can do about it with a goal to consume less processed and fast foods and more fresh whole foods including plenty of fruits and vegetables. The entire focus of the anti-inflammatory diet is health and healing your body's ailments.

This book also navigates through and beyond misinformation and myths surrounding the diet and lays the groundwork for your new lifestyle. It explains the variety of foods to eat for healing, what foods to avoid, and the best ways to cook meals to get the most benefit. In the end, you'll be equipped with the information you need to get started and to noticeably feel better including a one-week meal plan to get you on track.

There are plenty of books on this subject on the market, thanks again for choosing this one! Every effort was made to ensure it is full of as much useful information as possible, please enjoy!

Thanks,

Jason

Chapter 1: Why the Typical American Diet Is So Bad

Statistics available through the U.S. Department of Health & Human Services (HSS) shine a light on how bad the typical American diet is for us. For starters, "it exceeds the recommended intake levels or limits in four categories: calories from solid fats and added sugars; refined grains; sodium; and saturated fat." All this directly affects your health. In fact, the HSS says that "if Americans reduced the sodium they eat by 1,200 mg per day" going forward "it would save up to $20 billion a year in medical costs." We now get an astonishing 63% of our calories from refined or process foods. And while we eat too much of those foods, on the other end of the spectrum, Americans don't consume the recommended amounts of fruits, vegetables, whole-grains, and healthy oils. In fact, only 12% of our calories coming from plant-based foods. When you look at that statistic even closer, it's even worse because half of that already-low percentage comes from French fries. That means the real number of *healthy* plant-based foods is reduced to 6%, a figure that can only be described as horrifyingly low.

According to the HSS, calories containing no nutrients coming from solid fats and added sugars in the typical American diet "contribute to 40% of the total daily calories for 2 – 18-year-olds and half of these empty calories come from six sources: soda, fruit drinks, dairy desserts, grain desserts, pizza, and whole milk." Forty percent of daily calories! This means almost half of their daily calories contain little or no real nutrients because they are derived from these solid fats and added sugars. And what about the rest of us? Out of a 2775 daily calorie diet, the USDA estimated that in 2010 nearly 1,000 calories a day come from added fats and sweeteners, while only 424 calories came from dairy, fruits, and vegetables.

To better understand what we are talking about, it helps to understand that solid fats are fats that solidify at room temperature. This includes fats like butter, shortening, and fats that cook off of beef, pork, and other meats. Solid fats can be added when foods are processed by manufacturers or when they are prepared for consumption in restaurants or home. In the same way, added sugars include various types of sugars and syrups which are added when foods or beverages are processed or prepared.

In the last 65 years, the amount of sugar we consume has radically gone up, and along with that, the origin of where we get the sugar has also drastically changed. In the 1950s, Americans mostly ate sugar derived from sugarcane and sugar beets, but the year 2000, the USDA reports that each individual in America took in 150 pounds of sugar a year with more than half of that coming from corn in the form of high fructose corn syrup. And no, just because it comes from the plant corn does not make it a sweetener that's good for your health.

Over the last century, our palates have transformed along with the ingredients in our food. Just look at the ingredients list on the foods you buy. Ingredients are listed in the order of prevalence, with ingredients added in the greatest amount listed first, followed in descending order by those in smaller amounts. Sugar in one of its forms is often listed in the first three, because today with the typical American diet everything we eat needs to be really sweet, including foods we don't typically consider sweet such as bread. While sugar is needed to get the yeast to activate and ferment, if you check the label on that multi-grain bread, each slice provides 2.6 grams of sugar from honey and refined sugar.

What's more is, as you read the product label, sugar can be listed by numerous names. These names include anhydrous dextrose, cane juice, corn sweetener, corn syrup, dextrose, fructose, high-fructose corn syrup, corn syrup solids, invert sugar, malt syrup, maltose, lactose, sucrose and white sugar. Unfortunately, food manufacturers aren't required to separate added sugar from naturally occurring sugar but are only required to divulge total over-all sugars per serving.

With the consumption of all these empty calories, today more than 1 in 3 adults suffer from pre-diabetes. This condition happens as the result of higher than "normal" blood sugar levels which aren't at levels bad enough to be identified as type 2 diabetes. Plus, 30 million Americans are inflicted with diabetes but 1 out of 4 aren't even conscious of it.

The bottom line is that Americans aren't taking in enough vital nutrients, fiber, and natural fats needed to attain the best health. This is really sad when you think about how prosperous this great country is and yet we experience higher rates of disease than other developed nations.

What's the cumulative effect of the typical American diet over time? In a nutshell, the standard American diet can lead to chronic inflammation which leads to progressive tissue damage and inflammatory diseases like rheumatoid arthritis and leaky gut. Others ailments include what is known as "unexplained symptoms".

These include things like headaches, brain fog, bleeding gums, allergies, fatigue, mood swings, and skin rashes. In other words, random aches and pains that you can't identify the cause of. In the following chapters, we will take a closer look at chronic low-grade inflammation and what it does to the body. What does this all mean for you? Well simply put, many of your health problems could be caused by nothing more than the food you put into your body on a daily basis. Along with things like causing joint pain, it could well be the reason you're struggling with your weight!

Chapter 2: What Is Chronic Low-Grade Inflammation and Why Does It Make You Fat?

Chronic pain is a growing problem in America. People struggle to get through the day as they battle conditions like arthritis, fibromyalgia, back pain, and more. Many seek relief through strong prescription medication and while this may offer relief, it may also result in unwanted side effects. For those who would rather find another answer, a more natural answer, it's key to understand the connection linking inflammation and pain and the food we put in our mouth. Diets full of things like gluten, trans-fats, pasteurized dairy, corn (including corn sweeteners), and soy are at the source of the pain and inflammation – the same inflammation causing other medical conditions including overweight and obesity.

If you're battling your weight, even though you've cut calories, are exercising regularly and have stopped eating after 8 p.m., have you wondered why you're still carrying all that extra weight around your middle? It just might be that as hard as you are fighting to lose that excess weight, your body is fighting to keep it. Why? Chronic, low-grade inflammation caused by what you are eating.

To understand what one has to do with the other, first, we have to understand chronic inflammation. It is your body's bewildered and detrimental immune response to your environment. Which including poor diet, stress, allergens, and toxic substances. Research shows that what we eat is a significant contributor to chronic inflammation and our gut health. Other factors that contribute to chronic inflammation include a sedentary lifestyle and chronic stress, and living with hidden infections (including things like gum disease).

All these factors trigger this unseen inflammation running deep within our cells and tissues. Think of it like a smoldering fire and when we eat the wrong foods, all we're doing is feeding that fire. And when cytokines that respond to this unseen inflammation fill the bloodstream, it can lead to systemic inflammation, which in turn can lead to cardiovascular diseases. Cholesterol deposits cling to the lining of inflamed blood vessels and grow with a fatty plaque which can lead to blockages and blood clots which in turn can lead to a heart attack.

In this book, we will focus on the dietary link to inflammation, because over time, the continual inflammatory response to our diet is what can lead to weight gain and digestive issues. HHS reports that it is projected that "by 2030, half of all adults (115 million adults) in the United States will be obese." While normal inflammation is a good thing that works to protect and heal your body, chronic or systemic inflammation happens when your immune system gets out of balance and instead of healing, it contributes to disease and weight gain. The sugar we eat contributes to this shift in balance but it isn't the only culprit. Eating the wrong oils and fats including processed seed- and vegetable oils like soybean and corn oil, and hidden food allergens also contribute to the problem.

The influence of food allergens is the culprit directly related to weight gain. We're not talking about life-threatening food allergies some people have to specific foods like peanuts or shellfish, but is a different kind of reaction called a *delayed allergy* (IgG delated hypersensitivity reaction). This kind of deferred response may result in symptoms within a few hours or can be delayed for a few days after eating. This is a much more common allergy and leads millions of people to suffer because it plays a big part in numerous chronic ailments as well as problems with weight. In fact, it's a major contributor to obesity.

So, if you are on the older end of middle age or younger and struggling with your weight even though you think you're doing all the right things, then chronic inflammation could be the cause and an anti-inflammation diet the answer. Eating anti-inflammatory foods eliminates foods containing hidden food allergens and sensitivities, and can help you lose that stubborn weight effectively and permanently as long as you continue to eat the right foods.

Chronic inflammation wears down your immune system over time because it is on-going. As your body continually responds to this inflammation, it eventually leads to chronic diseases and other health issues including:

- Allergies which contribute to sinus and nasal congestion, weight gain, fluid retention, fatigue, joint pains, acne, eczema, brain fog, irritable bowel syndrome (IBS), mood issues, headaches

- Arthritis

- Asthma

- Autoimmune diseases

- Cancer

- Osteoporosis

- Premature aging

Regrettably, most often these chronic health challenges are treated with drugs and/or surgery, which may or may not offer temporary relief from symptoms, but these solutions don't actually address the root of the problem. But if you shop for the right doctor, today you can find an integrative MD who is willing to not only identify health issues but to address them by taking into consideration your lifestyle for ways to eliminate behaviors that lead to chronic inflammation. You can even ask them to run a CRP (C-reactive Protein test) to test your blood for a C-reactive protein which is a blood test marker for inflammation. It forms in the liver and is classified as an "acute phase reactant," which means levels grow higher in as a result of inflammation.

Chapter 3: Anti-Inflammatory Myths

While you can find plenty of information about eating to reduce inflammation, you'll also find plenty of myths and misinformation surrounding the anti-inflammatory diet, too. These myths include warning about foods to avoid as well as foods to eat, along with general all-encompassing statements like everything on the diet tastes terrible, or it's too expensive, so it's important to be informed so you don't sabotage your efforts toward better health before you really get started.

The myths listed in this chapter are deemed so because there's no scientific evidence to support them.

Myth #1: Citrus Fruits Bring About Inflammation

The need to ban citrus fruits because they cause inflammation is one of those unsubstantiated myths circulating on several online forums. The chatter condemns this fruit with little to no scientific evidence to back up claims. In truth, citrus is loaded with vitamin C and proven to reduce the progression of Osteoarthritis. Vitamin C is a beneficial antioxidant and citrus is also known to play an important part in the formation of cartilage.

Myth #2: A Raw Food Diet Alleviates Inflammation

While eating more fruits and vegetables is a good direction to go, eating an all-raw diet isn't necessarily the best solution to fight inflammation. A sudden change in diet like going all raw can actually help promote inflammation instead of relieving it, and the bacteria in your gut may have trouble processing foods so far out of your normal range of choices.

Myth 3: Gin-soaked Raisins Ease Symptoms

This myth is an old wives' tale that finds its origins in the hype surrounding the healing properties of juniper berries which are used to make gin combined with the belief that the sulfur in raisins eases joint pain. And while there may be an inkling of truth in this, it is an unrealistic claim because the amounts typically eaten are so small they make no real impact on your inflammation affecting joints.

Myth #4: Eating a Diet High in Fish Is the Same as Taking AlphaFlex or Fish Oil Supplements

Sorry to say, diet alone can't take the place of AlphaFlex® or other anti-inflammatory supplements. Although the Omega-3's found in fish have anti-inflammatory properties, you would have to eat a large quantity of fish to try to match the anti-inflammatory power of a supplement but you couldn't do it. Plus, fish can also be high in mercury, and excessive consumption could lead to the potential of mercury poisoning.

Myth 5: Eating a low-acid diet helps avoid arthritis flare-ups

The thinking behind this myth says to avoid foods high in acid, like citrus fruits and tomatoes to minimize pain and flare-ups. The problem with this is that as you eat and drink gets balanced once it enters your stomach. The digestive system adjusts foods whether acidic and alkaline and neutralizes and supposed benefit or detriment based on those qualifiers. Plus, citrus fruits are high in vitamin C which works as an anti-inflammatory.

Myth 6: Making Healthier Choices Is Cost Prohibitive

And one more myth related to following the anti-inflammatory diet is that healthier choices are cost prohibitive. It is true that processed foods filled with added sugars and higher fat content do cost less monetarily than nutrient-dense whole fruits, vegetables, lean meats. In fact, fresh vegetable and fruit prices rose almost 120% from 1985 – 2000. With those kinds of statistics, it does seem like making healthier choices is just too expensive for some of us. But that's really not the case.

Findings in a recent meta-analysis by researchers at Brown University and the Harvard School of Public Health shine a light on just how much more expensive it really is to buy healthier food options. They crunched numbers from 27 previous studies and what did they find? The cost for an adult to eat healthy comes to $1.48 a day more than eating a poor-quality diet. That calculates out to $550 more per person a year. Isn't that worth it for better health?

There are a few ways that can help you save more when eating a healthy anti-inflammatory diet. One of the big ones is to eat out less and to cook for yourself more. For instance, people spend an average of $11 per meal eating lunch out, but only $6.30 on average when they prepare their own lunch, plus when you make your own food you have the added benefit of knowing exactly what is in it. Also, as you increase the amount of fruits and vegetables in your diet, you'll find if you buy them in season you'll get the best value.

One last myth worth mentioning, even though it doesn't have anything to do with food and nutrition, is that *all anti-inflammatory medications have minimal side effects*. Sadly, the opposite is true. Even anti-inflammatory over-the-counter drugs like ibuprofen, naproxen, Celebrex and other non-steroidal drugs can result in a number of side effects, plus these drugs really need to be taken in prescription doses to curb inflammation.

These possible side effects include ulcers that may possibly become life-threatening, abdominal pain, diarrhea, dry mouth, kidney failure, swelling, and dizziness. On the flip side, fish oil is a natural supplement that fights inflammation without any known adverse side effects.

When searching for a fish oil, you should choose one that has the optimal EPA/DHA ratio. Ideally you want a supplement with 180mg EPA and 120mg DHA per serving.

Chapter 4: Top 7 Foods to Avoid

When eating to reduce inflammation, it is best to avoid most packaged foods because they contain inflammation-triggering preservatives, colorings, and artificial flavorings to increase their shelf life. If it is packaged in a box or bag, chances are that it's not good for your health. Eating too many inflammatory foods can lead to chronic low-grade inflammation which in turn can cause serious health issues including cancer, heart disease, diabetes, and allergies. With that said, this chapter looks at seven specific inflammatory foods to avoid.

1. Gluten and Wheat

As we've already discussed, inflammation is the natural response of your immune system. When we get a splinter, inflammation makes the surrounding area red and tender. With this picture in mind, let's look at why you should avoid gluten.

Proteins found in wheat are gut irritants, and the term "gluten" is a general name for these proteins. Now, picture tiny splinters raking into the lining of your gut and resulting in inflammation. When it comes to gluten, the most well-known gluten-related inflammation is celiac disease or non-celiac gluten sensitivity, but wheat can also be a problem for people who aren't specifically sensitive to gluten because of amylase trypsin inhibitors (ATIs) found in wheat. These ATIs can bring about an inflammatory immune response in the GI tract which contributes to another problem called intestinal permeability, or leaky gut, which we will cover more in chapter 8. This condition lets undigested food particles, bacteria, and toxic waste products "leak" through the intestines into your bloodstream.

2. Refined Carbohydrates

Carbohydrates are commonly referred to as "good" and "bad." Complex carbs are *good* because they are filled with beneficial fiber. When it comes to inflammation, refined carbohydrates fall into the bad category because in the refining process most of their fiber is removed. With the fiber removed, refined carbs raise blood sugar levels and raise the occurrence of inflammatory changes. This influence can lead to disease. For instance, when looking at our modern diet, research has shown refined carbs can encourage the development of inflammatory bacteria in the gut which can raise the probability of obesity and IBS.

3. Milk Lactose

Milk lactose is a sugar found in milk which causes digestive issues for many people because their bodies don't produce the lactase enzyme required to digest it. Other people who do produce this enzyme may still react poorly to drinking milk because of the proteins casein and whey. Casein actually has a molecular structure very similar to gluten, and half the people who can't tolerate gluten don't tolerate casein well either. As a result, dairy is one of the most inflammatory foods in today's diet, second only to gluten. Adverse digestive symptoms resulting from this inflammation may manifest in bloating, constipation, diarrhea, and gas. Other non-digestive symptoms include acne and a compelling demonstration of autistic behaviors. So lactose is only half the issue when it comes to milk and milk products, the others are the casein and whey proteins.

A study also showed that women in China have a far lower rate of breast cancer than women in the West. The only noticeable difference between the two diets is lower milk intake. A Harvard professor has also discovered links between ovarian cancer and dairy consumption.

4. **Sugar**

It's no secret that eating too many added sugars and refined carbohydrates can lead to overweight and obesity, but the consequences of eating excesses are also linked to increased gut permeability, raised inflammatory markers, and high LDL cholesterol. The thing all these factors have in common is that they can trigger low-grade chronic inflammation. Excess body fat, especially belly fat, results in continuous, chronic levels of inflammation which can modify how insulin works. Insulin, as a regulatory hormone, plays a big part in carrying the glucose in your bloodstream into your cells for energy, but when blood glucose levels are chronically high, the production and regulation of insulin is changed resulting in insulin resistance. The resulting overabundance of blood glucose can lead to an accumulation of advanced glycation end products (AGEs). When too many AGEs bind with our cells and integral proteins, it can lead to oxidative stress and inflammation. It can change their structure, inhibit their regular function and eventually result in a buildup of arterial plaque and decreased kidney function, among other things.

5. Meat

Grain fed beef has been touted as tasting better, but cows are naturally grazers that eat grass. When fed grain they grow fat quickly before they are sold by the pound for profit. Cattle, pigs, and chickens are not naturally grain eaters. But in life on the feed-lot not only are they fed things like corn and soy, they are also given antibiotics to make sure they don't get sick. This translates to meats on our dinner table that are not only higher in inflammatory saturated fats but also contain higher levels of inflammatory omega-6s from their unnatural diet. To compound the problem, when we grill our meat at high temperatures, it results in inflammatory carcinogens! So if you plan to eat meat, choose grass-fed varieties.

.

6. Saturated Fats

When you think saturated fats, many people think of red meat, but aside from fatty cuts of beef, saturated fat is also found in pork and lamb, the skin of chicken, as well as processed meats. It's also found in dairy products like butter, cream (including whipped cream), cheese, and regular-fat milk. Studies have linked the consumption of saturated fats with causing the kind of body fat that stores energy rather than burns it. As these fat cells grow bigger they release pro-inflammatory drivers that promote systemic inflammation.

7. Alcohol

Drinking alcohol puts a burden on the liver, and when consumed in excess, it weakens liver function. This disrupts other multi-organ interactions resulting in inflammation. If you choose to drink alcohol, do so in moderation, but it is best eliminated if you're fighting inflammation.

Chapter 5: Most Beneficial Foods and Best Anti-inflammatory Supplements

Many conditions can be traced back to inflammation. Joint pain, autoimmune disorders, irritable bowel syndrome (IBS), mood imbalances, acne, and eczema are just a few conditions that can be linked back to inflammation. Once the origin of inflammation is identified, an anti-inflammatory diet can help ease symptoms and certain foods and supplements can help lessen the inflammation in your body. In this chapter, we'll list some of the best minerals and beneficial antioxidants found in foods and supplements to add to your arsenal to fight inflammation. This list is arranged in alphabetical order to make it easier to use as a reference tool.

Blueberries

Blueberries make the list as an antioxidant superfood. This dark, delicious fruit may be small, but it's crammed with antioxidants and phytoflavinoids. These tiny berries are high in potassium and vitamin C and work as an anti-inflammatory to aid in lowering the risk of heart disease and cancer. They also assist with preventing mental decline. Strawberries, raspberries, and blackberries also contain anthocyanins which provide anti-inflammatory effects.

Avocado

Avocados are packed with potassium, magnesium, and fiber. This savory fruit is another superfood rich in antioxidants and anti-inflammatory properties. They provide a great source of healthy unsaturated fat and are packed with potassium, magnesium, and fiber.

Coenzyme Q10

Coenzyme Q10, also known as CoQ10, is another antioxidant that shown to offer anti-inflammatory properties. It is found naturally in avocados, olive oil, parsley, peanuts, beef liver, salmon, sardines, mackerel, spinach, and walnuts.

Ginger

Ginger is comparative to in that contains powerful anti-inflammatory compounds known as gingerols. Ginger root is found in the produce section at your grocery store and is available as a potent antioxidant supplement that helps prevent the oxidation of a damaging free radical called peroxynitrite. Ginger adds flavor to your favorite stir-fry, can be made into ginger tea, or can be taken as a supplement.

Glutathione

Glutathione is another antioxidant that fights free-radicals with anti-inflammatory properties. This is available as a supplement and is also available naturally in plant foods including apples, asparagus, avocados, garlic, grapefruit, spinach, tomatoes, and milk thistle.

Magnesium

Magnesium is a mineral supplement that can help reduce inflammation for those with low magnesium which is linked to stress. Statistics suggest an estimated 70% of Americans are deficient in this mineral which is surprising since it is readily available in a number of foods including dark leafy greens, almonds, avocado, and many legumes.

Salmon

Salmon is rich in anti-inflammatory omega-3s. It is better to eat wild caught than farmed. It is best to try to include oily fish in your diet two times a week, and if you're not a fan of fish, then try a high-quality fish oil supplement.

Turmeric/Curcumin

Turmeric is the yellow spice that gives curry its color, and curcumin is the active ingredient in turmeric and can be purchased as a supplement. The two words are often used interchangeably, but curcumin is the key ingredient which offers powerful anti-inflammatory effects. It's a strong antioxidant and as a powdered spice, turmeric can be added to soups and curries, and curcumin can be taken in supplement form.

Vitamin B

People with low levels of vitamin B6 have a tendency to have high levels of C-reactive protein which, as was mentioned in chapter 2, is a measure of inflammation in the body. B vitamins, including B6, can be found in vegetables like broccoli, bell peppers, cauliflower, kale, and mushrooms. It is also available in meats including chicken, cod, turkey, and tuna.

Folate (B-9 in natural form) and folic acid (a synthetic form of B-9) is another B vitamin linked to the reduction of inflammation. A brief Italian study submits that even daily, short-term low dosages of folic acid supplements can lessen inflammation in overweight people. Folate is found in foods like asparagus, black-eyed peas, dark leafy greens, and lima beans.

Vitamin D

Estimates suggest two-thirds of the people living in the U.S. are deficient in vitamin D. It's another vitamin that helps reduce inflammation, and getting insufficient amounts is linked to a range of inflammatory conditions. This vitamin is unique in that we get it naturally when we spend time in the sunshine with the important spectrum is ultraviolet B (UVB). It is also available as a supplement and is available in foods like egg yolks, fish and organ meats, as well as foods that are supplemented with it. When choosing a Vitamin D supplement, look for Vitamin D3, which is the most bioavailable form of the vitamin. The ideal amount for supplementation is 5000IU per day, and many of this pills cost less than $7 for a 3 month supply.

Vitamin E

Another potent antioxidant, this vitamin can aid in lessening inflammation. It is available as a quality supplement or can be found naturally in nuts and seeds, and vegetables like avocado and spinach.

Vitamin K

There are two kinds of vitamin K: K1 and K2. K1 is found in leafy greens, cabbage, and cauliflower. K2 is available in eggs and liver. This vitamin helps reduce inflammatory markers and may help to fight osteoporosis and heart disease.

Chapter 6: How to Extract the Most Nutrients from Your Food When Cooking

For decades, raw foodists have warned that cooking not only kills vitamins and minerals in food but also denatures the enzymes that help us digest the foods we eat. We've heard this for so long, many of us had embraced it as fact, but the truth is raw vegetables aren't always healthier, and in some cases, cooking is actually important if we want to get the most nutritional benefit from the foods we eat. Cooking can help us digest food without spending volumes of energy and makes foods like cellulose fiber and raw meat softer for and easier for our digestive systems to handle.

It turns out that vegetables like asparagus, cabbage, carrots, peppers, mushrooms, spinach, and numerous others, actually supply our bodies with more antioxidants like carotenoids and ferulic acid when boiled or steamed as opposed to raw. A January 2008 report in the Journal of Agriculture and Food Chemistry reported that when cooking vegetables "boiling and steaming preserved antioxidants better than frying." This was mainly the case with carotenoid present in broccoli, carrots, and zucchini. And before you shrug it off and say, "Any cooking method is better than frying," it's important to note that researchers actually examined the effect of several cooking methods on compounds such as carotenoids, polyphenols, and ascorbic acid and determined boiling to be the best way to extract these nutrients for consumption.

In the same year, a study published in The British Journal of Nutrition backed up this cooking benefit claim. This study consisted of a group of 198 participants and found those who adhered to an inflexible raw food diet showed normal quantities of vitamin A and comparatively elevated levels of beta-carotene. However, they had low levels of the antioxidant lycopene, a carotenoid with anti-inflammatory properties. Remember, these are findings for eating raw. In contrast, another study published in the Journal of Agriculture and Food Chemistry found that cooking essentially raises the quantity of lycopene in tomatoes. "The level of one type of lycopene, cis-lycopene, rose 35% after being cooked for 30 minutes at 190.4 degrees Fahrenheit." The conclusions drawn suggest that heat causes the thick cell walls of the plant to break down which aids in the body's absorption of nutrients which were bound to those cell walls.

So now that we know some nutrition is enhanced by cooking but not everything is best cooked, it leaves us with the question: "What should I cook and what should I eat raw on the anti-inflammatory diet?" The fact is that each food is a little different. The raw foodist mentality holds that many foods high in antioxidants are sensitive to cooking because phytonutrients don't hold up well to high temperatures and when it reaches the "heat labile point" it results in a change that causes foods to lose enzymes beneficial to us. But this is only half the story. The truth is that whether you should eat a vegetable cooked or raw for the most nutritional benefit depends on the vegetable and the way you cook it.

The hidden dangers of microwaving

Before we go any further, let's be clear – deep frying offers no benefit, and microwaving your food can actually bring about an inflammatory response. This is because microwaving brings about a change in the chemical structure of your food. In fact, it so completely alters the protein structure of food that the body doesn't even recognize it as a food, but instead looks at as a foreign toxin which warrants an inflammatory response.

Microwaving food is also harmful to nutritive benefit and leads to a loss of up to 90% of the nutritional value. It converts tasty, organic vegetables into nutritionally "dead" food that can bring about disease because microwaving changes plant alkaloids into carcinogens. I ake garlic for example. It's a powerful healing food when eaten raw and is of great benefit to digestive health, cellular immunity, heart health and more, but when microwaved for just 60 seconds the active component, allinase, become inactive. So the very component known to help protect against cancer is no longer any benefit at all.

The same kinds of changes occur when microwaving grains and milk, too. In these cases, the amino acids are converted into carcinogenic substances. When it comes to prepared meats microwaving again results in the development of cancer-causing agents. And if you use the microwave to thaw frozen fruits, it causes the sugar molecule to break down into carcinogenic substances.

An additional concern deals with carcinogenic toxins which can leach out of plastic containers, lids, or wraps used when microwaving. One of the nastiest contaminants is BPA which can cause chaos with our natural hormone levels. Often, BPAs can overstimulate the manufacture of oestrogen which can lead to oestrogenic cancers. So the next time you think about popping your food into the microwave, remember that microwaving results in molecular damage which not only kills nutritional benefits, but in its wake, leaves carcinogenic substances. So while it can seem convenient to rapidly heat your food, microwaving is not worth the nutritional loss or risk to your health.

Cooking with light heat or steam is the best as it breaks down food making it release easier-to-absorb nutrients. In some cases, as we've seen, it can even increase the nutrient content available. Another benefit related to cooking is that it can also transform chemicals from being potentially harmful to harmless. But, it depends on the vegetable and the method of cooking.

With all this in mind, the following list of vegetables is the ones better eaten cooked.

Asparagus:

The best way to cook asparagus is to steam or blanch it or bake it in a casserole. The process breaks down the fibrous spears making them easier to digest and allowing easier absorption of nutrients including vitamins A, B, C, E, and K.

Broccoli:

Finding the best way to cook broccoli is a little trickier. Those who have hypothyroidism, shouldn't eat your broccoli raw because it contains a thyroid-disrupting element. Steaming lets you preserve the nutrients while leaching out some of this element. Also, to retain a healthy amount of beneficial elements of broccoli, it helps to chop it before steaming. Avoid microwaving or boiling.

Carrots:

Carrots are best cooked by roasting or steaming. As the study mentioned earlier revealed, cooking your carrots can significantly raise the bioavailability of beta-carotene which is converted to vitamin A in our bodies. When you eat carrots raw, it's not absorbed as well.

Red Peppers:

When preparing red peppers roasting is the most advantageous. These vegetables are a remarkable source of carotenoids. And, like carrots, cooking can enhance the bioavailability of these carotenoids. However, don't overcook because it can destroy heat-sensitive antioxidants.

Spinach:

Dark green spinach leaves make a popular salad choice, but it turns out this is another vegetable that is better eaten cooked. Nutritionally, it's best to steam it. Because it wilts when steamed, one cup steamed holds more actual spinach as well as nutrients than one cup raw. But there's another cooking benefit related to the oxalic acid found in spinach. Oxalic acid hampers the absorption of certain minerals including calcium and iron and can even develop kidney stones. But cooking spinach reduces oxalic acid by 5—53%, and if you boil it, the percentage lost rises to 30—37%. However, steaming is better unless you are prone to kidney stones because boiling leaches folate from spinach leaves. Spinach is also advisable if you have a history of heart disease in the family.

Tomatoes:

Tomatoes are a rich source of lycopene which offers both anti-inflammatory and antioxidant properties and it, too, becomes more bioavailable after cooking. Just cook them with a little olive oil, or reduce tomatoes down to a sauce, tomato puree, or ketchup to notably increase the absorption of lycopene.

Chapter 7: Foods You Wouldn't Have Thought Were Good for You

It isn't uncommon when starting a diet to think, you'll have to give up everything you like, but with the anti-inflammatory diet, you may be pleasantly surprised to find there are delicious anti-inflammatory food and drinks options on the menu that you wouldn't have thought good for you.

Dark Chocolate

Let's start with chocolate. It not only makes for a special treat, it is actually good for you! When choosing chocolate with anti-inflammatory benefits look for chocolate that contains at least 70% cocoa (at the minimum). Along with being loaded with antioxidants that reduce inflammation, it may also lead to healthier aging because the flavonoids found in dark chocolate modify the production of a pro-inflammatory cytokine. Research suggests eating dark chocolate regularly or even occasionally can bring about beneficial results on blood pressure, oxidative stress, vascular damage, and insulin resistance.

Coffee

More than half of people in the United States drink coffee every day, but should we? Turns out coffee is actually the chief source of antioxidants in American diets. So it's okay to look forward to that cup of coffee in the morning for more than one reason whether it's decaf or regular because it contains polyphenols and other anti-inflammatory compounds. Numerous studies back this up, but one published in 2015 discovered that "over 30 years, nonsmokers who drank 3 to 5 cups of coffee a day were 15 percent less likely to die of any cause compared to people who didn't drink coffee." The coffee drinkers showed lower rates of death from heart disease, stroke, and neural conditions.

However, there is a downside to drinking coffee for some people as it causes some to experience insomnia, anxiety, irregular heartbeat and other negative side effects like irritation of the digestive system. If you experience any downside to drinking coffee, then it is best to avoid it. Try tea instead.

Tea

Green tea is another good-for-you beverage option. Of the many green teas available, Matcha tea is the most nutrient-rich. It offers up to 17 times more antioxidants than found in wild blueberries, and seven times more than what is in dark chocolate. What may surprise you, though, is that green, white or black tea all enjoy potent anti-inflammatory benefits. So if you're not a fan of green tea, you can drink the tea of your choice and still get the potent anti-inflammatory benefits of catechin polyphenols.

Garlic and Onions

Garlic and onions bring plenty of flavor to the anti-inflammatory food palate. Garlic has a long history as a staple folk treatment for colds and other illness. It provides sulfur compounds that encourage the immune system to battle disease. Garlic has been shown to work in the same way as over the counter nonsteroidal anti-inflammatory pain drugs like ibuprofen, by reducing pathways that lead to inflammation.

Onions provide comparable anti-inflammatory compounds, one of which is the phytonutrient quercetin, which breaks down to create free radical-fighting sulfenic acid. Crushing and chopping garlic and onion releases the enzyme alliinase, which helps form a nutrient called allicin. When consumed, allicin helps form other compounds that may protect us against disease.

Fermented Foods

If you're new to fermented foods they open a whole new experience in taste. Kombucha is a fermented lightly sweetened effervescent drink that's fermented. It's made with black or green tea and boasts a host of health benefits. You can buy kombucha in the cooler section of many stores, or if you're a DIY person, you can buy a kit or active Kombucha Scoby and you're your own. Along with kombucha, fermented dishes or products to try include kefir, miso, and sauerkraut. These cultured foods provide healthy bacteria which will optimize your gut health and support a healthy immune system, which in turn helps to reduce inflammation in the body.

In some ways, learning to follow an anti-inflammatory diet is a journey as you unlearn past behaviors and reinvent your tastes as to what is really good. Keep nuts like nuts like almonds and walnuts on hand for a go-to snack along with a selection of fruits like strawberries, blueberries, cherries, pineapple, and oranges.

Strawberries in particular are great if you're searching for a flat stomach. These delicious berries are packed with polyphenols which a study by the Texas Women's University found decreased the formation of fat cells in the stomach by up to 73%.

Yes, making changes to avoid inflammation does take some work and a change in thinking, and in some cases a change in the preferences of your taste buds, but when you realize you can enjoy foods you really like that actually heal your body and improve your health and even your mood and can save you money on drugs, you'll embrace the change.

Chapter 8: Healing Foods for Leaky Gut, Arthritis, and Other Associated Disease

We've talked about how the anti-inflammatory diet is a healing diet and, in this chapter, we will take a closer look at what that really means for people with leaky gut and arthritis. For many of us, looking at inflammation as a root cause is a new concept, because traditionally modern medicine treats it as a symptom. For instance, we know arthritis is inflammation of the joints. The common answer is to take medication to reduce inflammation, but that's only treating the symptom and isn't really addressing the real problem – what's causing the inflammation. When health professionals discuss an anti-inflammatory diet, this type of low-grade, chronic inflammation is what they normally expect to help.

Before we take a closer look at arthritis and what anti-inflammatory foods to eat to specifically to help combat that condition, we will discuss another condition that can leave you feeling depressed, fatigued, anxious, struggling with weight problems or digestive symptoms. We're talking about leaky gut syndrome which is also identified as increased intestinal permeability. It's a dangerous health condition in which your digestive tract gets damaged and permits bad bacteria, proteins like gluten, and undigested bits of food to pass into your bloodstream. Some of the early symptoms of leaky gut can include skin conditions like acne and eczema, food allergies, and digestive issues including bloating, gas and irritable bowel syndrome (IBS). Over time leaky gut causes systemic inflammation and an immune reaction. It's been associated with chronic diseases and conditions including asthma, autism, chronic fatigue syndrome, depression, diabetes, heart failure, IBS, infertility, kidney disease, lupus, multiple sclerosis, narcolepsy, psoriasis, rheumatoid arthritis, and more.

Most people don't begin to understand the role our intestines play in our overall health. The small intestine absorbs the majority of the vitamins and minerals from the foods we eat. For this absorption to take place, the small intestine is equipped with tiny pores that allow nutrients to be transferred into the bloodstream. The bloodstream works as a conduit that carries and deposits these nutrients around the body. Because the intestine has these tiny pores, the wall of the intestine is referred to as semi-permeable because it permits specific things like nutrients and other beneficial molecules to enter the bloodstream while blocking things like toxins and undigested food particles.

An unhealthy small intestine suffering from leak gut no longer works properly because the pores widen and allow harmful things to pass into your bloodstream and to be transported throughout the body. Often the body starts to recognize certain foods as toxic which results in an immune reaction every time you eat that food. If the problem goes on unchecked, leaky gut can advance to an autoimmune disease. To repair this increased intestinal permeability specific diet changes must be made.

Foods to Eat to Support Healing Leaky Gut

Foods that help leaky gut are easy to digest and can aid in healing the lining of the intestines:

Bone broth: Delivers important amino acids and minerals that can aid in healing heal leaky gut and improve mineral deficits. Best if made from scratch.

Probiotic-rich foods: Raw cultured dairy products like yogurt, kefir, and amasai can help heal the gut by wiping out bad bacteria.

Healthy fats: Consume healthy fats found in foods like avocados, egg yolks, coconut oil, salmon, and ghee in moderation. These fats promote healing and are easy on the gut.

Fermented vegetables: Foods like sauerkraut, kimchi, coconut kefir, or kvass contain probiotics vital in mending leaky gut by balancing the pH in the stomach and small intestines.

Steamed vegetables: Steamed non-starchy vegetables are easy to digest and a crucial part of the leaky gut diet.

Fruit: Fruit should be eaten in moderation; 1-2 servings each day. Best to eat it in the morning.

Foods to Eat to Support Arthritis

When the body is inflamed, C-reactive protein levels (CRP) rise, so if present it's a clear indicator of inflammation. Doctors can order a test checking for CRPs. According to studies published in *Molecular Nutrition & Food Research* and in the *Journal of Nutrition*, whole grains such as brown rice, bulgur, quinoa, and others have been linked with reduced CRP levels. Another study in the Journal of Nutrition discovered that people who ate smaller amounts of whole grains essentially experienced higher inflammation markers. According to the Arthritis Foundation, the fiber available in whole grains like oats can help resolve inflammatory processes by helping to achieve weight loss and by nourishing valuable gut bacteria linked with lower levels of inflammation and help soothe IBS. What we eat can make a difference in the inflammation associated with arthritis.

Types of Anti-inflammatory Foods to Eat to Help Arthritis

Foods Rich in Omega-3: Wild-caught fish, including salmon, is your best choice for omega-3 fats. Other foods to include in your diet include chia seeds, flax seeds, grass-fed beef, and walnuts.

Foods Rich In Sulfur: Sulfur boosts antioxidants and can help repair joints. Foods rich in sulfur include broccoli, brussels sprouts, cabbage, cauliflower, chives, collard greens, garlic, onions, garlic, grass-fed beef, leeks, organic eggs, radishes, raw dairy, watercress and wild-caught fish.

Bone Broth: Bone broth also makes the list for your arthritis diet because of its remarkable healing properties. According to nutrition researchers from the Weston A. Price Foundation, bone broth contains chondroitin sulfates and glucosamine which are the very compounds available in costly supplements designed to decrease joint pain and inflammation.

Fruits and Vegetables: Like every anti-inflammatory diet, fruits and vegetables are an important component. They provide digestive enzymes as well as anti-inflammatory compounds. When it comes to arthritis two of the best to be sure to include in your diet are papaya, which contains papain, and pineapple, which contains bromelain which research has shown may aid in decreasing disease-causing inflammation with ailments like rheumatoid arthritis.

Chapter 9: Anti-Inflammatory Herbs

Chronic inflammation is long-term. It results from the failure to eliminate whatever is causing the original acute inflammation and can last for months or even years. When people have inflammation, it often results in pain because of biochemical progressions that occur during inflammation leading to swelling that presses against sensitive nerve endings. This influences how nerves behave and can enhance pain. As a result, the kind of pain varies from one person to another and might come in the form of stiffness, discomfort, and even agony, but the thing sufferers have in common is that the pain is constant. It might be described as steady throbbing, stabbing, or pinching. Symptoms of chronic inflammation present in a number of ways including abdominal pain, chest pain, fatigue, fever, joint pain, mouth sores, muscle weakness and sometimes pain, and rashes.

Because of the side effects associated with traditional painkillers, many are turning to more natural herbal methods for healing and pain management. We've mentioned a handful of herbs and herbal supplements in earlier chapters, but here we dedicate the entire chapter to anti-inflammatory herbs. However, before you include herbal supplements in your health regime, it is best to talk with your doctor or pharmacist regarding any possible interactions with prescription or over-the-counter medications you may be taking.

Cayenne pepper:

The health benefits of cayenne and other hot chili peppers have been recognized since ancient times. Natural compounds called capsaicinoids are found in cayenne and all chili peppers. It's what gives them their spice and anti-inflammatory properties.

Black pepper:

The sharp taste of black pepper makes it one of the most popular spices in the world, but the piperine compound that gives black pepper that taste so many love is also a compound that prevents inflammation and makes it effective in reducing symptoms of arthritis.

Cinnamon:

Cinnamon is a common but popular spice often used to add flavor baked treats, but studies have shown it offers so much more than good flavor. This spice is rich in antioxidants, helps the body fight infection, and has anti-inflammatory properties which can ease swelling and repair tissue damage. Sprinkle it in your coffee or tea for a touch of flavor as just one way to enjoy its healing benefits.

Cloves:

Cloves are a pungent spice known for its anti-inflammatory properties. Researchers at the University of Florida conducted a study that had participants consume cloves daily and found that in just seven days it significantly lowered one specific pro-inflammatory cytokine. Because of its strong flavor, cloves pair well with nutmeg and cinnamon to add a tasty kick to stews and means. It's also a popular addition to Indian cuisine.

Devil's Claw:

This herb originally comes from South Africa and has been a remedy for African and European traditional and folk doctors used for centuries to treat digestive problems, relieve pain, reduce fever, and to treat some pregnancy symptoms. It also goes by the names wood spider or the grapple plant and it makes a popular choice for people suffering from arthritis and other forms of joint or back pain when combined with bromelain. In supplement form, devil's claw is derived from the dried roots of the plant. Research has shown it may have anti-inflammatory properties.

Ginger:

We talked about ginger as a supplement in chapter 5, but garlic in its natural form has been used for hundreds of years to treat things like constipation, sinus congestion, indigestion, colic and other digestive problems, as well as rheumatoid arthritis pain. When taken orally, garlic is said to be beneficial for helping with pain and arthritis. Cloves can be eaten raw or cooked, or it can be purchased as a supplement in powdered form in capsules or tablets. It's also available in liquid extracts and oils.

Rosemary:

Rosemary leaves are often used in cooking, but this herb is much more than an aromatic plant. It provides a whole range of possible health benefits. It's plentiful in antioxidants and anti-inflammatory compounds believed to aid in boosting the immune system.

Sage:

The medicinal use of sage goes way back. In the past, it's been used for ailments ranging from mental disorders to intestinal and digestive discomfort. In more recent years, studies show the health benefits of sage have grown since then. Not it appears to contain a range of anti-inflammatory and antioxidant compounds and research has reinforced some of its medical applications. Along with use in cooking, it is commonly used to make sage tea as a way to enjoy its many benefits.

Spirulina:

Spirulina is a blue-green algae and considered a superfood. It's a rich source of vitamin B12, full of antioxidants, and is approximately 62% amino acids. Research has established that Spirulina prevents the production and release of histamine, which is a chemical that kindles an inflammatory response in the body. Additional research confirms that Spirulina may lessen arthritis. However, Spirulina is not recommended for those who suffer from digestive issues because it is very difficult to digest.

Chapter 10: Start Feeling Better Instantly

Since we've covered how inflammation works, the health problems surrounding chronic inflammation, and the foods to eat to combat those problems, in this chapter we will discuss the benefits associated with eating a more plant-based diet along with other lifestyle aspects needed to help fight your way back to good health.

Growing evidence shows diet and lifestyle can either generate a pro-inflammatory environment or an anti-inflammatory environment. So, if you are suffering from chronic inflammation you can quickly start feeling better than you do at this moment by making lifestyle changes right now. The first step in is to start choosing the right foods, but it's more than that. Buying the right foods won't make a difference if you don't prepare them correctly. For that reason, it's just as important to learn how to prepare those foods using anti-inflammatory cooking methods (see chapter 6). If you don't, you can undo the very healthy benefits you're hoping to enjoy.

Remember, your daily food selections are the source of your chronic inflammation. To jumpstart your anti-inflammatory diet, embrace a more plant-based diet because when it comes to fighting chronic inflammation, one of the biggest benefits of consuming a plant-based diet is its ability to lower chronic inflammation levels. In fact, it is suggested that inflammation might just be the biggest reason why plant-based diets have been shown to promote health while our typical American diet promotes disease. To be clear, "plant-based" doesn't necessarily me no meat, because it can allow for limited quantities of fish and lean meat. What it does mean is a diet heavy in nutrient-dense vegetables and fruits that can aid in warding off inflammation and disease. In 2014 study on diet and inflammatory bowel disease, 33% of the participants in the study opted not to go with the proposed anti-inflammatory diet. The participants who did decide to follow the anti-inflammatory diet experienced enough relief that they could discontinue at least one of their medications.

Nutrient dense foods offer high levels of vitamins, minerals, and/or protein per serving. If you want to jumpstart your anti-inflammatory diet to start feeling better faster, along with buying and preparing nutrient-dense foods and preparing them properly, it's also important to stay hydrated, but to keep costs down your should drink tap water instead of bottled - unless you cannot drink the tap water in your area. Avoid chlorinated, waters because you're working to eliminate substances you don't need in your body. Staying hydrated helps to suppress cellular inflammation and will decrease inflammation in the body.

Along with taking care of what you put into your body, it's also important that you get regular adequate exercise. Doing so can actually boost your immune system. Not being active enough is actually hard on your body, but be careful to not overdo it. Plan 20-30 minutes of light to moderate exercise most day. With physical activity comes free radical damage and the breaking down of body tissue. This results in some low-level inflammation in the body as it heals during the recovery time between active times. So the goal is to find the middle ground. To be active, but not overactive. To move enough, but to rest enough. If you don't do this, it can result in inflammation to build up.

As the repairing and restoring process works within the body while you sleep, it's hard at work. For this reason, getting enough rest is important with doctors recommending 7 to 8 hours of sleep per night. If you're lacking in sleep, you're taking advantage of your immune system. As a result, it needs to work harder to try to keep you well. Lack of sleep leads to stress. Constant stress produces more cortisol and you guessed it, inflammation. So as you work to eat right, you need to put in the effort to also be active enough and to get your rest. It really is a lifestyle.

Chapter 11: Anti-inflammatory Meal Plan for 1 Week

As you reach toward better health going forward, your new goal is to consume a variety of nutrient-dense whole foods that can reduce inflammation. Making this move doesn't have to be hard, and it doesn't have to be expensive. You have plenty of foods to choose from and when you buy fruits and vegetable in season you will often find they cost less than a dollar per serving. The following list offers examples of anti-inflammatory foods that cost under a dollar per serving using in-season produce prices.

- Apples: $0.75 each

- Broccoli: $0.50 per 1/2 cup, $1.99 per bunch

- Cage-free Eggs: $0.25 per egg based on $2.99 a dozen

- Canned salmon: $0.80 for 4 oz. serving, based on $2.50 for 14.75 oz. can

- Cantaloupe: $0.50 for 1/2 cup, $3 per small melon and in season you can find them for much less

- Carrots: $0.50 each at $2 per pound

- Chicken breast: $0.75 for a 4-ounce serving, $2.99 per pound

- Garlic: $0.30 per bulb

- Grapes: $0.75 per cup, $1.50 per pound

- Kiwi: $0.40 each

- Mandarin oranges: $0.23 per piece, $3.99 for 5 pounds

- Onions: $0.18 each, $0.59 per pound

- Whole grain oats: $0.13 per serving, $3.98 for 30 oz. container. You can find oats for even less if you buy in bulk.

When you stop and really consider how many servings you get for your money when buying healthy foods, cost shouldn't really be a deterrent.

Sample Meal Plan for One Week

Day 1

Breakfast: Scrambled eggs served with chopped cabbage and onions seasoned with cumin seeds and turmeric. Steam until cabbage is softened but lightly crisp.

Lunch: Grilled salmon served on a bed of spring greens with olive oil and vinegar.

Dinner: Chicken breast seasoned with fresh herbs, and zesty lemon, steamed broccoli, and a serving of steamed brown rice.

Snack: 1 cup frozen grapes

Day 2

Breakfast: Oats (high in fiber, low in fat, oats contain *avenanthramides* which play a role in reducing inflammation). Add fruit like sliced banana or fresh dark-colored berries and a handful of walnuts.

Lunch: Spiced lentil soup seasoned with cinnamon, cayenne pepper, cumin, turmeric, and cayenne pepper

Dinner: Salmon patty (made using canned salmon, eggs, garlic, shallot, ginger, coconut flour, walnuts, cumin, turmeric, salt, and pepper), garden salad, topped with your favorite anti-inflammatory dressing.

Snack: Turmeric Chai Chia Pudding (from The Blenderist)

Day 3

Breakfast: Poached eggs served on fat-free refried beans topped with fresh salsa with sliced avocado on the side.

Lunch: Blueberry Banana smoothie made with coconut water and frozen banana

Dinner: Chicken curry made with sweet potato, broccoli, and cauliflower

Snack: Cup of diced cantaloupe

Day 4

Breakfast: Savory oats seasoned with cinnamon, a touch of ground coriander, ground cloves, ground ginger, a sprinkle of nutmeg and ground cardamom. Drizzle with a little real maple syrup which has a molecule with anti-inflammatory properties.

Lunch: Roasted sweet potato cut into strips like fries and served with avocado dip for a surprisingly delicious pairing

Dinner: Roasted garlic salmon with steamed cauliflower

Snack: Bell pepper strips with guacamole

Day 5

Breakfast: Pineapple smoothie made with green tea, kale, pineapple, frozen mango chunks, a tsp. of fresh ginger, and a pinch of turmeric

Lunch: Roasted red pepper and sweet potato soup

Dinner: Baked cod with pecan rosemary topping, and steamed green beans,

Snack: Cup of cherries

Day 6

Breakfast: Spinach and mushroom frittata

Lunch: Fruit salad made from your favorite in-season fruits

Dinner: Bell peppers, mushrooms, onions and diced tomatoes with chicken breast chunks, season with cayenne pepper for a little zip. Serve with quinoa

Snack: Dark chocolate

Day 7

Breakfast: Oatmeal seasoned with turmeric topped with plenty of colorful berries. Unique but delicious.

Lunch: Miso soup with gluten-free noodles

Dinner: Turkey and quinoa stuffed bell peppers

Snack: A serving of almonds

Conclusion

Thanks for making reading *Anti-Inflammatory Diet: Make these simple, inexpensive changes to your diet and start feeling better within 24 hours!*, let's hope it was informative and able to provide you with all of the tools you need to achieve your goals whatever they may be.

If the effects of chronic inflammation are robbing you of the joy of living because of pain, fatigue, weight gain or other health issues, it's time to take charge of your health. Now that you've read this book you are equipped to take steps toward healing. You've seen the statistics. Embrace the hope found in these pages and be proactive. Set a goal to consume less processed and fast foods and more fresh foods plentiful in fruits and vegetables. If you really want to see improvement, focus on health and healing, and that means thinking about every bite of food you take to get to your goal.

Don't be afraid to give up those favorite processed foods. They might taste good, but think about what you're really eating. Things like inflammation-triggering preservatives, artificial flavorings, and colorings, and then ask yourself if you want to still eat them. Don't think of it as depriving yourself, but instead think of it as empowering yourself to live healthier and pain-free. You don't have to be a slave to foods that aren't good for you, and you don't have to be controlled by pain or poor health.

Enjoy a piece of chocolate, and a cup of coffee and feel guilt free as you learn to eliminate inflammation triggering foods from your diet. You'll find a sense of freedom in just feeling better. Yes, it can take time, but remember it took time for the inflammation your fighting to become chronic. Each day is worth the fight toward better health, and now you have the arsenal at your fingertips to fight it.

Finally, if you found this book useful in any way, a review on Amazon is always appreciated!

Yours in health,

Jason Michaels

Anti-Inflammatory Diet: The Complete Guide for Managing Rheumatoid Arthritis and Healing Chronic Disease Using Healthy Food

By Jason Michaels

Introduction

Welcome, and thank you for being here.

The following chapters will discuss what exactly Rheumatoid Arthritis is, how someone can get it, and what happens when they do. More importantly though, we'll also talk about how an Anti-Inflammatory diet can help control and even reduce the effects of Rheumatoid Arthritis.

Rheumatoid Arthritis, can be painful, difficult, and lead to other diseases and conditions. There are medicines that you can take to help, but many times these medicines have terrible side effects, or can even cause worse things to happen.

Fortunately, there is another way. It's been shown that an Anti-Inflammatory diet actually helps and can even lessen the pain from Rheumatoid Arthritis. Your diet is arguably the most powerful natural weapon you have against this affliction. Which is why it's important to eat the right things and cut out all the foods that cause your inflammation to flare up. Specific foods can help with specific ailments; while it can be difficult at first to try and figure out what works and what doesn't, it's definitely worth it. In fact, there are even things you can do that other than a new diet to reduce inflammation! Managing your stress and being active really help to control inflammation, and this book includes different tips you can try that will help. These will be expanded on in the coming chapters.

Starting a new diet, in general, can be hard, and it makes it worse when you think you will have to cut out so many different foods from your life. Sometimes you're not sure where or how to begin! This book contains a sample menu for you to follow, along with recipes that only contains foods that can help to reduce your inflammation. You can use this information to jumpstart your new diet and get into the habit of eating healthy foods.

In addition to a new diet, you also have the option of using natural supplements. There are many supplements out there that can really help decrease your pain and inflammation, and they're definitely worth looking into if you want a potential alternative to pain medication. Not only will you learn which foods are best for you, but also which foods you shouldn't be eating.

Thanks again for choosing this book! Every effort was made to ensure it is full of as much useful information as possible, please enjoy!

Chapter 1: What is Rheumatoid Arthritis really?

Known by shorthand as RA, Rheumatoid Arthritis is a condition that attacks the immune system. Normally, the immune system of the body attacks unknown substances like viruses and bacteria as a way to try and stay healthy. This is why we tend to get a fever when sick; it's the body's way of telling us that it's fighting off the cold. However, those with rheumatoid arthritis deal with an immune system that makes the mistake of attacking the joints. When this happens, the joints become inflamed and the tissue lining the joints on the inside thickens. When the tissue thickens like that, it results in pain and swelling inside and around the joints. Normally the inside of the joints, called the synovium, creates a fluid that helps to lubricate them and move more smoothly. By thickening, the synovium can't create that lubrication. Think of it as oil inside a car. It's important to change your oil every few thousand miles, or else your car doesn't run smoothly. The tissue inside your joints acts the same way. By not producing "oil", your joints won't run as smooth as before.

Unfortunately, joint damage is irreversible. It's important to go to the doctor for an early diagnosis and treatment, otherwise, the inflammation can cause damaged cartilage and bones. Cartilage is the tissue that covers the ends of the bones in your joints. Without treatment, there becomes a loss of cartilage, and the space of the joints between the bones becomes smaller. When this happens, joints become unstable, painful, loose, and eventually lose their mobility altogether. The most commonly affected areas are the joints of the feet, wrists, hands, elbows, ankles, and knees. The effect is typically symmetrical; if one hand or knee if affected then usually the other one is as well.

Another reason that RA can be serious is that it can also affect your body's cardiovascular and respiratory systems. So not only are your joints affected, but also your heart and lungs! Around about one and a half million in the U.S. suffer from RA. It tends to show up in women more than men; three times as many women have RA as men. With women, it typically starts between ages 30 and 60, but with men, it usually occurs later in life. It's possible that having a family member with rheumatoid arthritis increases the odds of getting it yourself, but most people with RA don't have any family history of the disease.

There are specific goals with treating rheumatoid arthritis; stop inflammation, prevent joint and organ damage, reduce long-term complications, improve physical function and well-being, and to relieve symptoms. In order to meet these goals, your doctor will be following certain strategies. The first is early, aggressive treatment. The earlier, the better because you want to prevent any issues to your organs. The ultimate goal is to stop inflammation and achieve remission, which is when there is minimal or no signs of the inflammation being active. Doctors also want to achieve what's called "tight control', which is when they're able to get a disease to a low-level activity and keep it there. There are many medications that can ease symptoms and slow disease activity. There is also the option for surgery. But for those who don't want to use medication and surgery, there is the possibility of a specific diet helping, which is the Anti-Inflammatory Diet.

Chapter 2: How Do You Know You Have RA and What Comes With It?

It's possible you don't even realize you have Rheumatoid Arthritis. Maybe you're finding it harder and harder to get up in the morning. Maybe you're feeling stiff throughout your whole body that always seems to linger. It's possible this can be attributed to getting older, but what if there's something more serious going on?

Luckily, there are specific signs and symptoms that can tell you for certain if you have Rheumatoid Arthritis:

- You begin by experiencing a feeling of stiffness and/or joint pain.

- Your joints, and the area on your skin around your joints begin to turn red.

- The symptoms happen in at least four joints.

- These symptoms coincide with the opposite joint; they affect both the right and left side of the same joint. Basically, you can feel it in both hands, not just one or the other.

- When you first wake up for the day, you feel an overall stiffness throughout your body, and it typically lasts at least 30 minutes.

- If you have any of the above symptoms for a consistent amount of time.

While it's more than likely you'll experience the above signs, it's also possible to experience signs not directly associated with Rheumatoid Arthritis:

- You start losing weight and don't know why.

- You have a feeling of chronic fatigue that won't go away.

- You seem to have developed a low-grade fever.

- You have a feeling of depression that you're not able to get rid of.

- Your appetite changes.

- You seem to get sick on a regular basis.

Rheumatoid Arthritis can also affect non-joint structures within the body as well, including eyes, skin, nerve tissue, salivary glands, and other main organs.

The symptoms can vary in severity and it's even possible the signs just come and go. Flares or flare ups are moments that alternate between increased pain and no pain at all. You might think it just went away on its own, but that's not the case. In fact, RA has the possibility to make your joints move out of their normal area! It's very painful and requires going to your doctor.

There are specific facts that can increase the chances of getting Rheumatoid Arthritis:

Sex: women over men have a higher chance of developing Rheumatoid Arthritis.

Age: RA can happen anytime, but it typically starts between 40 - 60 years old.

Family history: it can be genetic; it's entirely possible that if a family member has RA, then you might have a greater chance of getting it too.

Smoking: smoking cigarettes increases the risk of you developing RA. Also, it's been seen that smoking is associated with an even greater severity of the disease.

Environment: it's also possible that your environmental exposure can increase the risk of Rheumatoid Arthritis. Asbestos, silica, and other unhealthy dust can create a higher risk for developing an autoimmune disease.

Obesity: people who are overweight or obese tend to be at more risk to develop RA, especially for women who have been diagnosed younger than 55 years old.

There is also the chance of developing certain complications when diagnosed with Rheumatoid Arthritis:

Osteoporosis: osteoporosis happens when the bones become weak, which puts them at a higher risk of fracturing. Rheumatoid Arthritis can increase your chance of developing osteoporosis, and unfortunately, some of the medications used for treating RA can cause it as well.

Rheumatoid nodules: nodules are little tissue bombs that are typically formed within the pressure points, like your knees. And while they are most commonly found there, they can be found all over the body, including important organs.

Dry mouth and eyes: those with Rheumatoid Arthritis are at risk to form a condition called Sjogren's Syndrome, which is a condition that dries out the moisture and wetness from your mouth/eyes.

Infections: unfortunately, Rheumatoid Arthritis and many of the different medications used to combat it can weaken the immune system, which in turn leads to an increase in infections.

Abnormal body composition: for those who have Rheumatoid Arthritis, they tend to have a higher fat proportion compared to their lean mass, even for those that have a typical BMI.

Carpal tunnel syndrome: this condition is commonly found in those who work at a computer all day; it affects your hands and wrists, causing them to hurt. Combined with Rheumatoid Arthritis, carpal tunnel feels much worse due to the compression of the nerves that serve your fingers and hands.

Heart problems: RA has a higher risk for blocked and hardened arteries, in addition to causing inflammation in the area that surrounds and the heart.

Chapter 3: How to use diet to increase your quality of life

When people hear the word "diet", they typically think of it as in the traditional sense, as a way to lose weight. Most diets are thought of as fads, and people usually stay on them for a specific amount of time. But the Anti-Inflammatory Diet isn't a normal diet and isn't intended as a weight loss program. It's a way of choosing and preparing foods based on scientific knowledge that specifically help with inflammation and maintaining optimal health. And not only does this diet help with inflammation, it also provides ample vitamins, energy, minerals, important fatty acids, and dietary fiber.

It's entirely possible that living an unhealthy lifestyle can cause inflammation to flare up. Processed foods have ingredients that are very unhealthy! Sugar, high-fructose corn syrup, and refined carbs can all lead to insulin resistance, diabetes, inflammation, and obesity. And eating processed food with trans-fat in it has actually been shown to trigger inflammation, in addition to damaging the lining of your arteries. Vegetable oils might seem healthy, but because they have an imbalance of omega-3s to omega-6s, they result in inflammation. Plus, excessive alcohol intake, processed meat, and an inactive lifestyle call all lead to inflammatory effects on the body.

The best way to counter all these bad foods promoting your inflammation is by changing your diet. It's important to eat nutrient-dense foods that contain antioxidants, which help to reduce molecules in your body that can possibly lead to inflammation. These foods include making the right proportions of fat, protein, and carbs for every meal. It's essential to remember to stick with healthy carbs and not processed refined carbs, like white bread. This is made easier by eating a lot of fruit and vegetables, but it's also important to remember to eat a variety of different things so you won't be bored with your diet.

An anti-inflammatory diet specifically can help Rheumatoid Arthritis; especially making sure to eat the foods that relieve the symptoms of RA. Fish oil especially can help with arthritic pain.

Anti-Inflammatory Diet Benefits for those living with RA

An Anti-Inflammatory Diet is based on the simple concept that out of control or continuous inflammation in your body leads to bad health and eating certain things that help to prevent inflammation can lead to better health and keeping the disease from affecting you.

It's even possible that illnesses other than arthritis can be triggered by inflammation; cancer, heart disease, diabetes, and Alzheimer's. Inflammation is actually natural and essential to the body healing itself, but it's only healthy when it happens only when needed. Chronic inflammation is when serious damage can be done.

So not only can an Anti-Inflammatory diet help with inflammation and the aforementioned conditions, but there are also many other benefits:

Better Brain: inflammation has been shown to cause an increase in feelings of depression. It contributes to mental exhaustion, indecisiveness, anxiety, and brain fog. As you now know, eating a lot of carbs, sugars, bad fats, and processed foods can cause blood sugar difficulties that result in insulin resistance, which can then result in diabetes. Eating these things can also increase body fat, inflammation, and depression. By taking away processed foods, high fructose corn syrup, sugar alcohols, refined sugar, and trans fats, you can actually achieve a more alert and better mental state. By replacing those empty calories with nutrients around in fruits and vegetables, you give your energy and brain a much needed health boost. It's not just fruits and vegetables though - protein in the form of organic meats, small fish, and pastured eggs contain good fat, which is something your brain needs to function well. This good fat "omega-3" is found in all these protein sources, so it's important not to skip them!

Glowing skin: Your skin can definitely be affected by what you eat. There are some out there that break out if they eat pizza sauce! It's more than just skipping the sauce on your pizza though. Inflammation and skin issues are actually directly related to each other. All those foods that cause inflammation - sugar, bad fats, processed foods - can cause skin problems like acne, blemishes, psoriasis, dullness, rosacea, rashes, and itchiness. Cutting out dairy, processed foods, and refined sugars can significantly improve the skin's appearance by getting rid of inflammation. And as an added bonus, the vitamins, minerals, and antioxidants found in fresh fruits and vegetables can make a person glow with amazingly healthy skin! Consuming foods such as coconut oil, seafood, turmeric, ginger, green tea, avocados, etc. can really help your skin to improve.

Weight loss: Getting rid of the main sources of allergies and food sensitivities like corn, dairy, gluten, nuts, and yeast products is the key to helping decrease inflammation and can lead to significant weight loss. Some people can also have strong reactions and inflammation when consuming nightshades, like peppers, eggplants, potatoes, tomatoes, and citrus, like oranges. The best way to figure out what causes your inflammation is by doing the elimination diet. Try the easy version first, by eliminating dairy, eggs, and gluten. If you still don't notice a decrease in your inflammation and weight, try getting rid of the rest of the food mentioned in your diet. The main reason an Anti-Inflammation diet helps with weight loss is that inflammation is one of the main factors in diabetes. When your fat cells become inflamed, there's the possibility of them creating insulin resistance, which is a predictor of possible future weight gain. And even worse, inflammation of the brain can cause "leptin resistance". Leptin balances out your metabolism and appetite, so when it's impaired then the metabolism is impaired, which then causes weight gain. Plus, inflammation decreases your insulin sensitivity, which has the possibility of leading to obesity, which in turn can lead to diabetes. So by going on an Anti-Inflammation diet, you're actually helping yourself become much healthier, and kick-starting your body into losing weight!

No more bloating: Dairy and gluten are major contributors to bloating, diarrhea, gas, and constipation. Definitely, something no one wants to deal with! This tends to happen with the bad microorganisms in your gut outnumber the good ones. Normally, your gut flora is there to keep out all the bad stuff so you don't get sick, but if your flora isn't working or is compromised, then bad bacteria can take up residence and inflammation follows. When you have sensitivities to certain foods, the bad bacteria is exacerbated and creates havoc in your gut. However, once you stop eating inflammation causing foods, your body begins the healing process and starts to rebalance the gut flora; typically this takes about 3 to 6 months. Probiotics and prebiotics can help even further to balance the gut. Probiotics help supply beneficial bacteria and can be found in either supplemental form or through fermented foods like kimchi, sauerkraut, and kefir. Prebiotic foods provide important nutrients that help to support good bacteria and can be found in artichokes, garlic, onions, and jicama. However, as a side note, if you have SIBO (small intestinal bacterial overgrowth), where bacteria moves into the small intestine where they shouldn't be, then you need to avoid probiotics because they'll feed the bacteria that has moved into your small intestine and make the issue even worse.

Cravings: Surprisingly, it's actually not normal to have intense food cravings. They're a sign that something is out of whack with your body, especially when you're craving sweets. Artificial sweeteners and refined sugars can create a terrible cycle of food cravings and inflammation that perpetuate one another because of chemical changes that occur in your body, especially in your brain and gut. And when your body is inflamed, eating foods like these will make the situation much worse. So the key to stopping this terrible cycle permanently is by getting your cravings under control. Which is easier said than done! There are several things you can do to combat the cravings and get them under control:

- Start your day with a good and healthy breakfast that contains proteins and good fats.

- Have proteins and healthy fats with every meal to balance your blood sugar.

- Eat regularly so your blood sugar doesn't drop, which incites cravings.

- Choose whole foods, especially leafy greens, vegetables, and fruits.

- Consume spices like cloves, cinnamon, cardamom, nutmeg, and coriander to naturally control your cravings.

- Deficiencies in nutrients can make your cravings worse, so it helps to take high-quality multivitamins and mineral supplements even while getting vitamins and minerals from your food sources. Specifically, chromium, magnesium, and Vitamin B3 can help to improve blood sugar control.

Joint pain relief: It can be annoying or even feel excruciating when you have inflammation in your joints. You end up feeling irritable and not really wanting to move or do anything. And while there are other factors to consider that contribute to your joint pain, what you eat and consume is often a significant source of inflammation. By altering your diet, you can actually eliminate your pain! Sugar and gluten are the two biggest contributors to inflammation and thus joint pain. Unfortunately, most people with chronic pain are addicted to sugar and carbs. And consuming it overruns the vegetables and fruit they eat, which are critical building blocks that cells need to make the body run healthily and properly. Replacing grain-based products and sugars with berries and vegetables, and removing gluten from your diet, can result in having a steady reduction of pain. After a while, the pain even fades completely away.

Say bye to autoimmune: It's very common to have some sort of autoimmune issue, but it's definitely not normal or healthy. Having this disorder can take a large toll on you; if you're diagnosed with one, you're familiar with the feeling of discomfort, pain, and helplessness that comes when trying to combat an autoimmune disease. But by changing your diet, you can actually decrease inflammation and flare-ups. A big impact on you feeling better quickly is phasing out inflammatory foods. Ingesting trigger foods like dairy and gluten can make your body react with joint pain, bloating, headaches, and GI distress. It's even possible for no symptoms to occur sometimes. When you eat those triggering foods, your body then creates inflammation and antibodies at the same time, which then triggers an autoimmune reaction.

A specific trigger in food sensitivity is gluten intolerance which can cause chronic inflammation and lead to an autoimmune disorder. Although, technically any food can cause inflammation, so it's important to do an elimination diet so you can find your own personal triggers. Eliminating gluten, eggs, dairy, grains, seeds, soy, citrus, tomatoes, nuts, potatoes, eggplant, and peppers are a great place to start when you have an autoimmune condition. Get rid of all of these from your diet, then add them back in one at a time after 8 weeks.

Take 6 to 8 weeks for each food item so you can specifically see and feel any changes from that one item. If certain foods cause any symptoms, then you need to completely avoid them. A healthy and beneficial protein is actually bone broth. It contains gelatin, which is made of the amino acids proline, glycine, and glutamine. These all help to reduce inflammation and help with having a healthy gut. Glycine specifically is known to help with hard to control immune activity. Besides gelatin, more helpful additives are olive oil, fish oil, flaxseed oil, and ground flaxseed. And although it's a little expensive, eating wild salmon at least 3 times a week can be extremely beneficial. All of these contain omega-3's which are extremely healthy and necessary for a good diet, while meat, poultry, egg yolk, and dairy fat all contain omega-6, which is the unhealthy fat.

Burn fat: Inflammation and obesity are almost always linked together since they both cause what's called "leptin resistance". Leptin is a hormone that's produced by body fat. It's there to tell your brain when you're feeling full and helps to lessen your appetite and increase your metabolism. However, if your body is leptin resistant, then those "feeling full" messages don't get to your brain and you find it difficult to actually feel full. Basically, it becomes incredibly easy to overeat. When someone is obese, the muscles, liver, and fat all stimulate inflammation, which promotes even more obesity and leptin resistance. It's a vicious cycle, and one that's hard to break free from. Back in the 90's, the "low-fat" fad started, and really changed the way people thought about foods they considered to be fatty. People ended up thinking the good fats were actually bad and tried replacing them with other fats that are actually bad! Anything with trans-fat, partially hydrogenated oils and polyunsaturated vegetable oils are all considered unhealthy, and shouldn't be a part of an actual healthy diet. Luckily there are healthy fats out there, and they're essential for balancing inflammation. Fats from coconut, olives, most nuts, avocado, and tallow are great and can actually help you to burn fat! By making these a part of your anti-inflammatory diet, you will end up feeling full more quickly, eliminate your cravings, and stabilize your blood sugar.

Allergies: Many people have a sensitivity to dust, mold, spores, and pollen. These are inhalant allergies and can cause sneezing, runny and stuffy nose, watery and itchy eyes, and a headache. For most, it hits in the springtime when pollen is in the air, and these seasonal allergies can drive someone crazy. Unfortunately, there are those that have allergy reactions year round; those that get irritated from mold and pets. If you get allergies from things in the air, whether seasonal or year round, it's entirely possible that you're sensitive to certain foods as well. When your gut is compromised from inflammation, you're more than likely to have in increase in allergy levels from eating certain foods. Basically, if you have inflammation, then you have a higher chance of getting a stuffy nose! So by removing foods that cause inflammation from your diet, your seasonal allergies could actually significantly decrease. Some example foods you can get rid of to help your allergies are: bananas, caffeine, red wine, white wine, beer, champagne, yeasty foods, pickles, soy sauce, fish sauce, citrus, fermented foods like kombucha, dairy, peanuts, food additives, dyes, processed meats, red meat, sugar, artificial sweeteners, and wheat.

Fatigue: Our adrenal glands are pretty important; they produce two key hormones that we need in order to live full and healthy lives. The glands sit on top of our kidneys and are responsible for producing the hormone aldosterone, which regulates blood pressure, and cortisol, which helps to manage metabolism. Adrenal fatigue can happen when your body is systematically inflamed, or when you eat a lot of carbs, refined sugars, and other inflammation causing foods. The most common symptoms to look out for are feelings of being overwhelmed, low grade depression, weight gain, fatigue, anxiety, and difficulty getting out of bed. You might feel tired, but as if you have a lot of spastic energy as well. It's possible for you to crave sugar in a feeling similar to addiction, and you can even develop a muffin top. Other symptoms include difficulty focusing, moodiness, skin inflammation, excessive hunger, irritability, and sugary/salty food cravings. If any of these symptoms seem familiar, or you suspect you're suffering from adrenal fatigue, you should consider doing an elimination diet. Try recipes and the meal plans outlined in this book and see if you're feeling any better. And although alcohol, caffeine, sugar, and gluten filled foods seem like a quick fix when you're feeling burnt out, it's much better to stay away from them. Consuming these will only make the issue worse and put further strain on your adrenal glands.

Chapter 5: Inflammation Causing Foods to Avoid

By taking away specific foods from your typical diet, you're actually making one of the best decisions possible to help reduce inflammation. Interestingly enough, the foods that cause the greatest inflammation are the ones with the highest risk of allergy and sensitivity. Example foods to avoid are:

Dairy: Lactose is an ingredient found in dairy and is a type of sugar that most have trouble digesting. Dairy also contains "casein", a type of protein that can trigger inflammation in most people.

Wheat: Many different types of wheat (bread, pasta, desserts, etc.) can cause inflammation in most people. Many have a sensitivity to gluten, which is found in all these products. Of course, it's possible to not have a gluten allergy or sensitivity, but the best way to find out is by doing an elimination diet, which is where you take away everything of a certain food for about 6 - 8 weeks, and then slowly reintroduce things one at a time. If you're feeling worse when eating products with wheat, but better without, then that might be a sign of gluten sensitivity. There are other options available, and in today's market, it's extremely easy to find pasta and bread that don't have gluten.

Eggs: Eggs happen to be in many different things, which means it can be difficult to determine if they cause any sort of reaction. Some people are allergic to just the yolk, and some just egg whites. The best course of action is to give up eggs and anything with egg in it (cakes, sauces, protein powders, baked goods, etc.) in an elimination diet.

Meat: Inorganic meat, or even ones that are advertised as corn-fed or vegetarian-fed. It can be difficult to find organic meat, but most local health food stores have them, or you can even check online. Inorganic meat contains large amounts of what's called "arachidonic acid"; something found in our bodies that can lead to inflammation, so too much of it in your diet can cause inflammation.

Processed Foods: Processed foods all contain sugar and corn syrup, which causes inflammation to happen. Avoid candy, soda, lunch meat, hot dogs, etc.

Nightshade Vegetables: Tomatoes, potatoes, eggplants, etc., all have what's called "solanine", which is a substance that has been found to cause inflammation and pain in many people.

Citrus/Tropical: There are some people who are sensitive to citrus and tropical fruits, like oranges, papayas, mangos, pineapples, etc. The best way to see if these fruits are affecting you is by cutting them out for 6 to 8 weeks and reintroducing them one at a time to see if you're being affected by a specific individual fruit.

Alcohol: Many alcohols have wheat in them and can cause inflammation. It's possible that red wine is fine to digest but try the cutting out and reintroducing test to find out for sure.

Specific Oils: Corn oil and soybean oil can cause inflammation and pain.

Basically, the best thing you can do is minimize or avoid completely foods with lots of sugar and sugary drinks, too much alcohol, and foods that have a lot of refined carbs and bad fats. If you're unsure about a specific food, then try removing it from your diet for 6 to 8 weeks and reintroducing it. It can be difficult and annoying to be constantly taking away and reintroducing foods but dealing with inflammation is much worse. And once you find out which foods are causing it, you'll be able to have a steady diet that really helps you to be your healthiest self!

Chapter 6: Foods to Eat

When switching to an anti-inflammatory diet, the most important thing to remember is eating the foods that can help. It might seem difficult at first, especially for those of us who have a sweet tooth! But there is actually a lot of different foods you can have, even sweet and tasty things. Fruit is a very good option when looking for something sweet and combining it with dark chocolate or unsweetened cocoa powder can make for a tasty treat!

Fruits/Vegetables: Fruit and vegetables that are locally grown, in season, and organic is best. One of the biggest things most people struggle with when eating organic is the cost. Organic food is more expensive, and most people just don't want to pay a ton of money for some apples or kale. Instead, try going to a local farmer's market! Fruit and vegetables there are fresh, organic, and typically much cheaper than store bought organic. It's basically cutting out the middle man and spending less money to be a lot healthier. Some good fruits to eat are grapes, cherries, strawberries, etc. And some good vegetables to eat are kale, broccoli, cauliflower, brussels sprouts, cabbage, etc.

Meat: Meat is on both the foods to avoid and foods to eat list. That's because while most meat isn't that healthy for you; organic lean meats are actually really good to eat! The best meat to choose is chicken, turkey, and fish, and make sure to choose organic kosher meat. Doing so will ensure that you're getting the best possible type of meat that won't cause inflammation.

Fish: Cold water and small fish are the best types of fish. They have low amounts of mercury and very high amounts of omega-3 fatty acids. Both of these can prevent inflammation.

Spices: There are actually spices out there that decrease inflammation. And not only can they do that, they're tasty too! Turmeric, ginger, and rosemary are a few examples of anti-inflammation spices. You can put them on many different things, and still be healthy.

Organic Beans/Whole Grains: Brown rice and quinoa are a couple of examples. You can experiment with making delicious soups and stews with any of these examples and try other ones as well. Soups and stews are great because you can make them in a crock-pot and freeze what you don't use for other nights. Making a big batch helps you to eat healthy on days you don't feel like actually cooking; instead just heat up what you already made! Beans and whole grains also have a wide variety of fiber and nutrients, which benefit in the aid of healthy digestion and lowering cholesterol.

Oil: cold pressed oils are best, like olive oil. They are processed less, so unlike margarine, they are more anti-inflammatory and better for keeping up with a healthy heart.

Blackstrap molasses: interestingly enough, there are many people with Rheumatoid Arthritis that swear by blackstrap molasses even though the actual scientific research is limited. The best answer that doctors can come up with is that this specific molass is full of nutrients and vitamins, including magnesium, which helps to preserve muscle function, nerve function, and joint cartilage. Low levels of magnesium tend to be more common in those with RA and can be a risk factor for heart disease. If you don't want to eat blackstrap molasses, maybe because of the unsure scientific research or that you don't like molasses, then you can instead consume nuts, beans, bananas, green vegetables, and whole grains.

Sour Cherries and Pomegranates: both of these fruits contain the flavonoid anthocyanin. Pomegranates, in particular, have many beneficial properties, including reducing inflammation. Sour cherries contain zashin, which helps with symptom improvement. They have large amounts of antioxidants and help keep your body healthy. Plus, sour cherries are low in nitric oxide, which interestingly enough, is connected to Rheumatoid Arthritis.

Parsley: not just a garnish, parsley actually can be very helpful in blocking inflammatory proteins. It contains the flavonoid luteolin, which is an anti-inflammatory that can help reduce stiffness and pain.

It can be difficult to switch to healthier foods, especially if your body isn't used to it. But anything can become a habit, even eating healthy! All of these options can help in preventing inflammation, reducing long lasting pain, and improve your health overall.

Chapter 7: 19 Mouthwatering Anti-Inflammatory Meals

The best meal plan for an Anti-Inflammatory diet incorporates many vegetables, fruits, whole grains, fish, and organic meat. It can be difficult to follow a strict meal plan when you don't have a clear idea of where to start or exactly what recipes to eat. One of the most important things you can do is meal planning; it and preparation are the keys to succeeding in any diet. One thing you can do that will really help is fill your fridge and pantry with just anti-inflammatory foods. By doing this, you don't automatically go for something unhealthy anytime you want a snack. It's definitely easier to munch on some chips or go through a drive through on the way home because you're just so hungry. But if you plan ahead, then you'll be less likely to do that, and you'll end up eating healthier! It's also important to figure out substitutes you can use instead of the unhealthy options. For example, instead of eating high-carb pasta, you can make zucchini or squash noodles. Instead of going straight for that bagel, invest in a blender to make yummy and nutritious smoothies!

Below is a sample menu that will hopefully give you some ideas of where to begin! By following these examples, you can start eating healthier and really begin to help your problematic inflammation. Follow these in order or try mixing and matching!

Breakfast: steel cut oats with blueberries; millet porridge cooked in coconut milk with mango and blueberries; cooked quinoa topped with raspberries and toasted walnuts; sweet potato pancakes with almond butter.

Lunch: sautéed mushrooms, kale, egg seasoned with turmeric with a pineapple ginger smoothie; Mexican chopped salad with creamy avocado dressing, with a pineapple ginger smoothie; large mixed greens salad with fried egg and a spiced banana almond smoothie; loaded baked sweet potato with a spiced banana almond smoothie; lentil veggie bowl; large salad topped with salmon cakes with balsamic dressing, and a pineapple ginger smoothie.

Dinner: Thai veggie curry stir fry with chicken; salmon cakes, broccoli, and a green salad; grilled chicken, sautéed spinach, and garlic green beans; veggie burger with a lettuce bun, baked sweet potato fries, small side salad; grilled salmon, asparagus, and potatoes, spring barley and quinoa risotto with asparagus and shiitake mushroom with chicken; quinoa stuffed peppers.

When you're not used to eating many vegetables, a sample menu like this can feel daunting! But if you're strict, and really stick to it, you could start to see results within weeks! If you're still feeling pain after following this menu, try taking out specific things, like meat, in an elimination diet. It's possible something very specific is causing your pain, so it could take a while to figure out which food you need to cut out altogether. You'll have to experiment a little but following this menu and the recipes in the next chapter is a step in the right direction.

Anti Inflammatory Shopping Checklist

Here's a specific shopping list you can use to make some stable recipes and get you started:

- Leafy green vegetables (spinach, kale, etc.)

- Olive Oil

- Tomatoes

- Lentils

- Whole Grains

- Fruits (blueberries, strawberries, cherries)

- Fatty Fish (salmon, mackerel, tuna, etc.)

- Turmeric

- Sweet Potatoes

- Shiitake Mushrooms

- Nuts

- Curry

- Cumin

- Beets

- Broccoli

- Chicken

- Cauliflower

- Chickpeas

- Carrots

- Celery

- Coconut Oil

- Ginger

- Raw Oats

- Fish Oil

- Berries

- Bok Choy

Quinoa and Turmeric Chicken

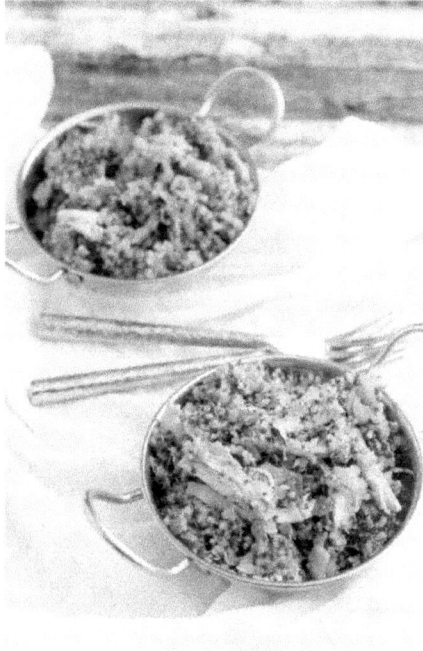

Ingredients:

2 pounds skinless boneless tempeh chicken

4 garlic cloves

1/2 t pepper

1 t salt

1/2 t cumin

1 T olive oil

1 T fresh ginger, grated or chopped

1 onion

1 t turmeric

1 1/2 t curry powder

2 plum tomatoes

2 c quinoa

2 bay leaves

2 3/4 c broth

1 1/2 T Asian fish sauce

Instructions:

1. Take the chicken, and season it with salt/pepper.

2. In a pan, heat oil to medium, put in the turmeric.

3. Place in chicken and stir.

4. Cooking time is when chicken on both sides is a little brown, then set aside.

5. Shred chicken once it's cooled down.

6. Put the ginger in the pan, along with the onion, for 8 mins of cooking time.

7. Add cumin, quinoa, garlic, and tomatoes, along with curry powder. Stir without stopping, 3 mins of cooking time.

8. Add in the bay leaves, along with the broth and fish sauce. Also, put in the shredded chicken. Heat up everything into the pot into a simmer.

9. You'll have 25 mins of cooking time, make sure to put a lid over the pan before starting the timer.

10.   Once time is up, take the pan off the stove. Keep it covered for 5 more mins, then enjoy!

Coconut Flour Pancakes

Ingredients:

1/4 c of coconut flour

1/2 t vanilla

1/8 t baking soda

1/3 to 1/4 c of coconut milk

Pinch of salt

3 eggs

2 T of coconut oil

1 - 2 T honey

Maple syrup to taste

Butter for cooking

Instructions:

1. In a bowl, combine together honey, eggs, and oil until blended well.

2. Add in the vanilla extract and coconut milk.

3. Put in the baking soda, salt, and coconut flour. Mix a little, but not too much.

4. In a pan, melt butter and put in a little batter. Keep in mind, the amount you use depends on how big you want your pancakes to be and how many pancakes you want to make.

5. Flip when ready.

6. Serve pancakes right away, added with maple syrup to taste.

Coconut and Sweet Potato Muffins

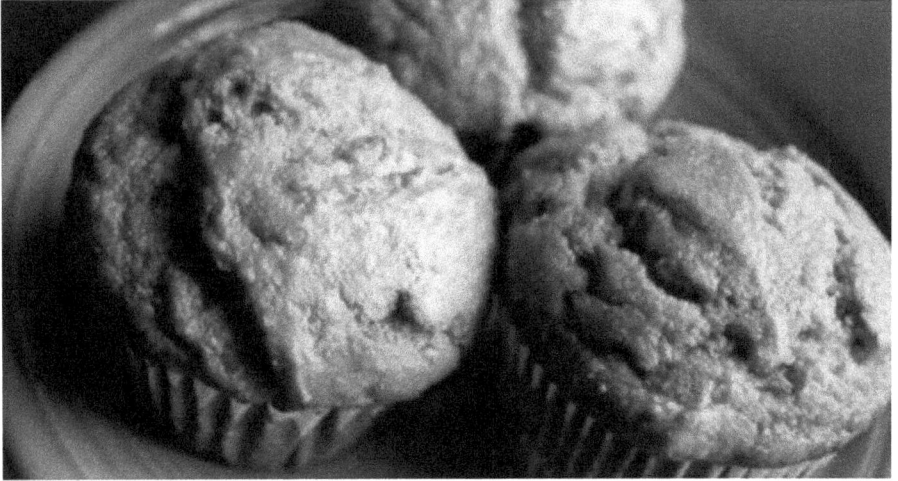

Ingredients:

3 eggs

1 small sweet potato, roasted

1 c brown rice flour

3/4 c canned coconut milk

2 T olive oil

1 c coconut flour

1 T of baking powder

1/2 t pink Himalayan salt

1 t ginger, ground

1 T cinnamon, ground

1/2 c maple syrup

1/8 t of nutmeg, ground

1/8 t of cloves, ground

Instructions:

1. Cook in the oven at 400 degrees F.

2. In the sweet potato, poke holes so it can cook all the way through. Put into oven, the rack that's in the middle is typically best for overall cooking. It cooks for 60 minutes of cooking time.

3. Take the potato out of the oven and set aside to cool down.

4. Once cool, take the inside of the sweet potato, peeling the skin off. Put the innards into a bowl.

5. In mixing bowl with the sweet potato, add olive oil, the beaten eggs, maple syrup, and the coconut milk. Mix until smooth.

6. Take a different bowl and combine all the other ingredients and mix well.

7. Mix all the ingredients together and stir to blend.

8. In an oiled pan (best if you use a muffin tin, but you can use a normal baking sheet if necessary), scoop the batter and fill every section about 2/3.

9. Muffins cook for 30 to 35 mins of cooking time. Place muffin tin in the oven, typically the rack in the middle is best for thorough cooking. To test when ready, insert a toothpick or knife into a muffin and make sure it doesn't have any muffin on it when you take it back out.

Curried Chickpea Lettuce Wraps

Ingredients:

Chickpea Filling:

1 onion

1 t turmeric

1 can chickpeas

6 mint leaves

1 T olive oil

1 t cumin

1 T sesame seeds

1 garlic clove

1 t ground chili peppers

1 T flax seeds

1 avocado

Salad:

1 avocado

1 garlic clove

1 t lime juice

2 tomatoes

1 spring onion

12 basil leaves

2 T crushed walnuts

1 pointed green pepper, chopped

6 lettuce leaves, washed

Instructions:

1. In a pan, put the chickpeas with around 1/4 c water. Put in the turmeric and chili powder. Stir to coat everything at about medium to high heat for 2 to 3 minutes.

2. When there is almost no water, add the rest of the chickpea filling ingredients (onion, garlic, olive oil, cumin, flax seeds, mint leaves, sesame seeds) and stir together for around 1 minute. Then turn off the heat and cover with a lid.

3. In a little bowl, smash the avocado and 1/2 chopped tomato. Put in lime juice plus minced garlic, and blend well by stirring. If needed, you can also use a blender to make it smoother. Add in the rest of the salad ingredients (garlic clove, spring onion, basil leaves, pointed

green pepper, and rest of the chopped tomato). Salt to taste and combine.

4. Top with the crushed walnuts.

5. Place 2 tablespoons of the chickpea filling into the middle of one of the lettuce leaves. Add 2 tablespoons of the salad. Repeat with the other lettuce leaves.

6. This recipe is best if eaten right away, but you can store the salad and chickpea filling in the fridge for at most 1 day.

Buddha Bowl

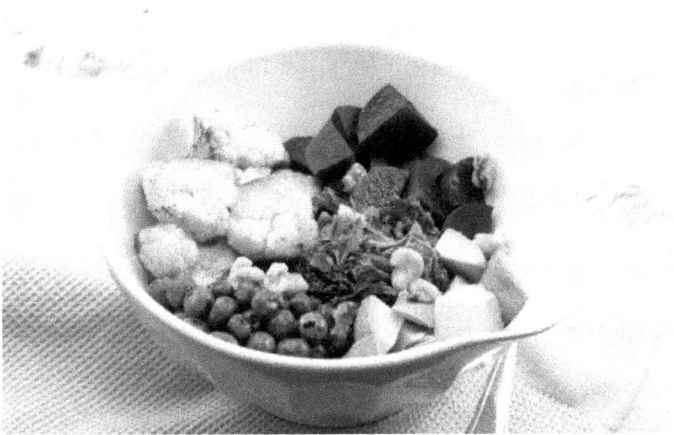

Ingredients:

2 pounds of cauliflower florets with stems removed and broken into chunks

1 t turmeric

10 ounces of chopped kale

1 T olive oil

8 medium cooked beets, peeled and quartered

2 avocados

2 c of blueberries

1 clove of garlic

1/3 c chopped raw walnuts

Salt and pepper as desired

Optional: cayenne pepper or nutritional yeast

Instructions:

1. Cooking temperature is set at 425 F.

2. Take a baking sheet, place foil on it, and put either olive or coconut oil, then leave it for later.

3. Toss cauliflower with olive oil in a large bowl.

4. Sprinkle turmeric over cauliflower and toss.

5. Spread out cauliflower on the baking sheet, and lightly sprinkle salt, pepper, cayenne pepper, and yeast.

6. Bake cauliflower for 30 minutes, check at 20 minutes.

7. While cauliflower is baking, heat a pan to a medium type heat with either coconut or olive oil.

8. Add kale to heated up pan and toss until the kale just about starts to wilt and grate in the garlic. Toss to coat.

9. Cut avocados into slices or chunks.

10.   Divide kale among the bowls, and top with the roasted turmeric cauliflower, beets, blueberries, walnuts, and avocados.

No Bake Sugar Free Apricot Turmeric Lemon Bars

Top tip: These are great to batch make to you can grab one on days where your body won't let you cook.

Ingredients:

1 c of oats

1/2 c walnuts

1 and 1/2 c of dried apricots

1/4 c lemon juice

Pinch of black pepper

1 t organic lemon zest, divided separately into 1 teaspoon and 1 teaspoon

1 t vanilla

1 T chia seeds

1 and 1/2 t turmeric, ground

1 T of the soaking water from apricots

1/4 c of shredded coconut (for dusting)

Additional topping ideas for variety, feel free to include all or none of the following:

Cacao nibs

Almond slivers

Crushed walnuts

Chia seeds

Pumpkin seeds

Instructions:

1. Take the dried apricots and soak them in hot water for around 5 to 10 minutes. Once they have softened, drain the water from them but keep 1 tablespoon of the water and set aside.

2. Place the apricots and all of the other ingredients into the food processor EXCEPT the reserved water, 1 teaspoon of the lemon zest, the coconut, and any of the other toppings you want to be included. Blend until the mixture is similar to a dough-like consistency.

3. If the mixture ends up being too dry, add in the reserved 1 tablespoon of water.

4. Use parchment paper to line an 8x8 dish. On it, scoop mixture press down firmly to evenly distribute the dough.

5. Top with the coconut, the remaining 1 teaspoon of lemon zest, and any of the other desired toppings.

6. Place in the refrigerator for at least 2 to 3 hours before serving so the bars can become more firm. The result, in the end, is supposed to be sticky and soft. Store the bars covered in the fridge.

Cherry Smoothie with Mango

Ingredients:

1/2 c of water

1 c mango, frozen

1 c sweet cherries, frozen

3/4 c water

Instructions:

1. Put mangoes plus the cherries into separate bowls to thaw. Usually takes about 10 mins to be ready.

2. Take cherries and the 1/2 c of water, put in a blender, and mix until well blended. Put in another 1/4 cup of water if the concoction seems thick. Once done, put the mixture into a separate cup.

3. Wash out the blender and put in 3/4 c water, in addition to the mango. Blend together well. Again, put in extra water if the mixture seems too thick. Take the mixture and pour it over the layer of cherry smoothie in the cup.

4. Drink up!

Turmeric Oatmeal

Ingredients:

Oatmeal

1 c of water

A little splash of milk that is plant-based

1/2 t turmeric

1/2 c of whole oats

Possible Toppings

Blueberries

Any berries you prefer

Any type of nut slivers

Any type of seeds

Desiccated coconut

Dried berries

Any type of syrup, maple tastes best with this recipe

Instructions:

1. Add in a pot and cook the oatmeal ingredients together (water, whole rolled oats, oat milk, turmeric powder) until the oatmeal is soft.

2. Place in bowl and top with either all or some of the toppings (blueberries, other berries, nut slivers, desiccated coconut, seeds, dried berries). Drizzle syrup over everything if desired.

3. Enjoy!

Cannellini Beans with Garlic and Sage

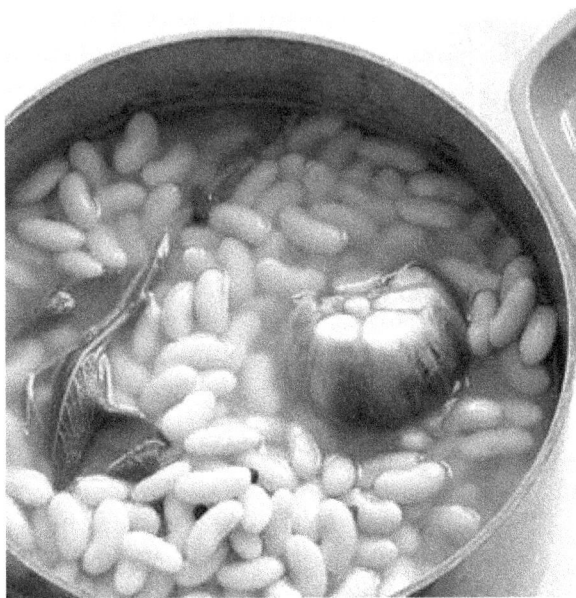

Ingredients:

1 lb. kidney beans also called cannellini

1 head of garlic that isn't peeled. Take off about a half inch at the top so the cloves are showing.

1/4 t whole black peppercorns

1 large fresh sage sprig

1 t salt, best is salt that is kosher and coarse

2 T olive oil

Extra virgin olive oil

8 c room temperature water

Instructions:

1. The first thing that needs to be done is soaking the beans overnight, so place them in a bowl. They need to be completely covered, so make sure there's at least one inch above the top of the beans.

2. The next day, the beans need to be drained. After you do that, put them in a pot, large is best.

3. Put in the 8 c of water, along with everything else except the salt.

4. Heat up the pot to a heat of about medium/high in a simmer.

5. Once you've reached the simmer, lower the heat and keep it there for around one and a half hours. Stir every once in a while to ensure maximum flavor.

6. After the 1 and 1/2 hours, stir in 1 tsp of salt. Keeping simmering for an additional 30 mins, or until beans are no longer hard. If needed, add more water to keep the beans covered.

7. Once beans are tender, take beans off heat and let cool for about an hour.

8. Take a spoon that has holes in it and move the beans to a different bowl. Taste is best if leaving the spices in the pot, which is why you use a spoon with holes.

9. Season with salt and pepper to desired taste, add a little bit of the oil on top, and enjoy!

Chicken Enchilada Cauliflower Rice Bowl

Ingredients:

Riced Cauliflower

1 chopped cauliflower (makes about 4 cups)

1 and 1/2 t of salt

Lime juice, about a medium's worth

2 T of cilantro

1 t chili powder

Chicken Enchiladas

Enchilada sauce, best if red and in an 8 oz can/package

2 t of chili powder

4 skinless boneless chicken breasts

Toppings

Grilled corn

Cilantro

Black beans

Olives, black ones are best

Tomatoes

Instructions:

Chicken Enchiladas

1. Mix together all the ingredients for the chicken enchiladas in a slow cooker (chicken, sauce, and powder).

2. Croc pots, or any slow cookers, take a while to actually cook something, so there's a window of 4 to 6 hours of cooking time. Make sure to place the lid on top and put it on the low setting. You'll know it's done when the chicken feels tender.

3. After the chicken is finished cooking, break it apart into shredded pieces of meat. This is easiest when done with a fork. After shredding, coat it with the sauce.

Riced Cauliflower

1. The first thing you need to do is rinse off the cauliflower. Make sure you get any extra stuff on there off, and once you do that, then use a paper towel to dry it.

2. Cut the vegetable in half and take out the middle core area. Then use the knife to cut the rest of it into large pieces, which then go into a food processor.

3. Blend it until it's around the size of couscous or rice. Usually takes about 15 pulses. You can also use a grater if necessary.

4. Heat up a pan to about a higher medium heat. Make sure it's coated with oil or spray before putting any food in it.

5. Once it's heated up, put the cauliflower, salt, and chili and garlic powders in the pan.

6. Sauté everything, cooking time is typically around 4 mins.

7. Put the lime juice into the concoction, along with the cilantro. It's only about 1 more min to be ready.

How to put everything together:

1. Place a little bit of the riced cauliflower in a bowl.

2. Take everything else, and place over the rice. Enjoy!

Lemon Basil Baked Salmon

Ingredients:

6 ounce filet Salmon, cut into 4 pieces

2 Lemons

2 T garlic

1/2 c butter

1 teaspoon basil leaf

A pinch of red pepper flakes

Foil

Oil to go into the pan

Instructions:

1. Cooking temperature is set at 374 F.

2. Lay out foil sheets, one for each filet, spray with cooking spray and place salmon on foil.

3. Combine butter, garlic, basil, and red pepper into the small pot. Keep on a lower heat. It's done when butter has melted completely.

4. Spoon butter mixture evenly over fish filets.

5. Squeeze half of a lemon over each filet.

6. Wrap up the filets into the foil and put them onto the cooking tray.

7. Bake 15 to 17 mins.

8. Turn oven on broil, set to high.

9. Broil 1 to 2 minutes to make the filet edges crispy.

10.   Serve immediately and enjoy.

Honey Sesame Seared Salmon

Ingredients:

2 to 3 pounds of salmon fillets

1/4 c of oil, best if using sesame

2 T of honey

1 lemon, juiced

1/4 c of coconut aminos

1 t ginger powder

1/4 t garlic powder

Coconut oil for searing

Diced chives to go on top

Some sesame oil to go on top

Some sesame seeds to go on top

Instructions:

1. Blend together until smooth everything except the salmon (sesame oil, coconut aminos, honey, garlic/garlic powder, ginger/ginger powder).

2. Take a bag that can seal, or you can use a glass dish, and place the filets into the bag (or dish, but it must have a top).

3. Put the sauce in the bag with the salmon. Place in the fridge. Marinating time is typically around 3 to 4 hrs., but you can leave it in the fridge overnight if you prefer.

4. When it's time to cook, take a pan or skillet, and heat it up to about a medium heat. Put in 1 - 2 tablespoons of the oil.

5. Put the fish in the pan, but make sure the side that is placed down is the one with skin. It should make a sizzling sound once you put it in the pan.

6. Cooking time is about 2 - 3 mins. Once time is up, turn the fish over to cook the other side.

7. Put in the whatever's left of the sauce and reduce heat to a lower setting. Cooking time is about 3 to 5 minutes, or until it's done.

8. Salmon will be done when you're able to use a fork and it flakes off.

9. Serve the cooked salmon with green onions, fresh chopped chives, sesame seeds and oil.

Thai Style Papaya Salad

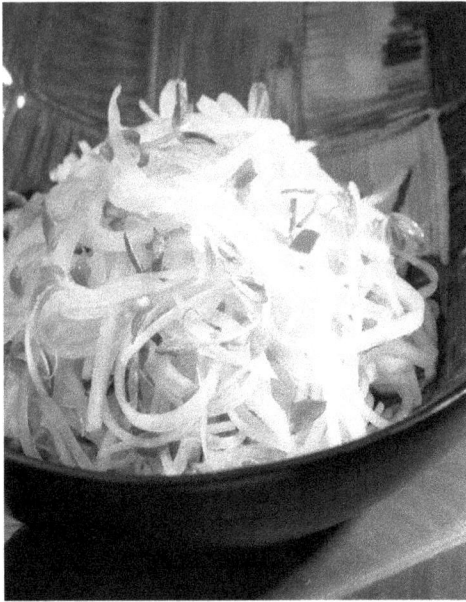

Ingredients:

2 T fish sauce

1/4 c of lime juice

2 T brown sugar, make sure the tbs are firmly packed

1/4 t freshly grated lime zest

3 c green papaya, cut into very small pieces

Hawaiian (or any fresh hot chilis) chilis, minced

1/2 c sweet onion, cut into very small pieces

1/2 c pea shoots, best if cut in 3 in sections.

Instructions:

1. In a bowl, mix lime juice, lime zest, chilis, and sugar. Along with the fish sauce.

2. Once you've added the previous ingredients, mix in the onions, papaya, and pea shoots into your bowl and mix them altogether by tossing. Dust lightly with the pepper to taste.

3. Enjoy!

Pomegranate Winter Salsa

Ingredients:

2 and 1/2 c of pomegranate arils

1 and 1/3 c of diced cucumbers, seeds removed

1/4 to 1/3 c cilantro

1/3 c of red onion, best if the onion is diced

A half of a lime, squeezed

1 to 3 jalapeños

Instructions:

1. Mix everything together, but make sure you start with the jalapeño first. Blend well by stirring.

2. If the combination isn't spicy enough, you can add in the extra jalapeños to make it as spicy as you'd like.

*1 jalapeño is equal to mild salsa, 2 jalapeños is equal to medium salsa, and 3 jalapeños are equal to hot salsa.

Quick Carrot Rice Breakfast

Ingredients:

4 t sweet tamari soy sauce

2-3 t molasses or coconut palm sugar

1 t water

3 garlic cloves

2 cayenne peppers or Thai red peppers

Pinch of ground ginger

1/3 c of small shallots (onion to substitute)

4 large carrots

1/3 c chopped broccoli

1 c bean sprouts

2 eggs

1 c ground cooked chicken breakfast sausage

2 T sesame or avocado oil

Salt and pepper as desired

Cilantro for garnishing

Instructions:

1. To make the sweet soy sauce: boil 1 tablespoon tamari, molasses, and water. Reduce until molasses is dissolved, set aside.

2. To make the spicy sauce: blend together cayenne pepper, shallots, ginger, and garlic. Set aside.

3. Rice carrots and broccoli.

4. Add spicy sauce to pan with oil, fry on medium heat until fragrant.

5. Add chicken sausage to pan.

6. Cook on medium high until cooked through, about 3-5 minutes.

7. Add eggs, fry together for 2 minutes.

8. Add rice carrots, riced broccoli, and bean sprouts.

9. Mix on medium heat.

10.   Add 3 tablespoons of tamari sauce. Add salt and pepper as desired.

11.   Time of cooking is 1 - 2 minutes until everything is coated.

12.   Serve into 2 to 3 bowls, add an additional fried egg on top of each bowl.

Chili Garlic Cauliflower Risotto

Ingredients:

Chili Garlic Cream Sauce

1 avocado, best is on the smaller side

1/2 c of either coconut or almond milk

2 to 3 t of minced garlic

1/2 t ginger

2 T of chili sauce or paste

1 t of red chili pepper flakes

A pinch of pepper to taste

1/4 t of salt, you can use sea salt if you'd prefer

1 to 2 T of honey OR agave

2 t of tamari that's gluten free OR gluten free Worcestershire sauce

Optional 2 tablespoons of water or oil to thin out the dressing

Cauliflower Rice Risotto

1 small head cauliflower (about 14 ounces)

1/4 c onion, yellow is best for this recipe

1 to 2 t olive oil

1/2 c of coconut milk

1 t of minced garlic

2 - 3 T bell peppers, color is your preference

1 small pepper, sliced

Cucumber slices for topping

1 bunch of basil, chopped

1/4 c toasted pumpkin seeds or nuts, crushed

Lemon or lime juice

Salt and pepper as desired

Instructions:

1. The first step is to make the dressing. Blend together the avocado, chili sauce, garlic, pepper, and coconut milk.

2. Add in the spices, Worcestershire/tamari, honey/agave, and ginger. If you want the sauce to be thinner, add in 2 to 4 tablespoons of water or coconut milk, along with a little oil.

3. Mix until the texture of the concoction is on the thinner side. Taste test and see how bitter it is, and if it's too bitter then add in a little extra honey.

4. Take the cauliflower and chop off the leaves and stems. You're left with the floret, and they need to be a similar consistency of rice, which is best done in a food processor.

5. Take out the riced cauliflower of the processor and set aside in separate bowl.

6. Take the oil, onion, and garlic and place in a pan. Sauté time is about 1 to 2 minutes.

7. Add in the cauliflower risotto rice and the red peppers. Cook time is 2 - 3 minutes.

8. Put in 1/2 cup of almond/coconut milk. If you'd prefer a creamier salad, add in 2 to 3 tablespoons of coconut cream or non-dairy milk.

9. Cook on medium heat, coating the cauliflower rice risotto. Also put in the pepper, salt, and a smidge of lemon juice.

10. Take the pan off the heat and place your riced cauliflower risotto into another bowl.

11. Top with chili peppers, sliced green bell peppers, crushed nuts, sliced cucumber, and chopped basil.

12. Drizzle the chili garlic cream sauce over each bowl once ready to serve.

13. Enjoy!

Chocolate Hazelnut Protein Cookies

Ingredients:

8 ounces of hazelnuts

1/2 c dark chocolate chips

1 banana

1/2 c coconut sugar

1 t vanilla

2 T coconut oil

Pinch of salt

1 T cocoa powder

1/2 c chocolate Vegan Protein Powder

Melted extra dark chocolate for topping

Extra hazelnuts for topping

Instructions:

1. Blend hazelnuts and chocolate chips together in a food processor until it represents a "mealy" base. It'll be a little moist from the chocolate.

2. Place base in a bowl.

3. Add in banana, coconut oil, and extracts. Beat until blended well.

4. Add in protein, sugar, cocoa. Mix until well blended.

5. Roll dough into small golf ball sized spheres. Place the dough onto a pre-greased cookie sheet. It's best if the dough is flatter on top, so you can use the back of a spoon.

6. Cooking temperature is 350 F, and time is 10 - 12 mins, or until cookies are a little browned at edges.

7. While cookies are cooling, drizzle the melted dark chocolate on top and add crushed hazelnuts.

8. Put cookies in the fridge for about 30 minutes to harden.

9. Enjoy!

Slow Cooker Jambalaya

Ingredients:

2 t seasoning, Cajun flavored

1 lb. of andouille sausage

2 t parsley

1 lb. black forest ham, cubed

1 c celery

1 onion

1 bell pepper

1 c broth, your preference

1 lb. of chicken breast, which needs to be cut into little 1 in cubes

2 t oregano

1/2 t dried thyme

Optional 1 t chili powder

Optional shrimp or crawfish, 1/2 to 1 pound

1 can diced tomato with juice, 28 ounce can

1 t of cayenne pepper

Instructions:

1. Chop onions, bell pepper, celery, and mix them plus everything else together into a slow cooker.

2. 7 - 8 hrs. is the typical measurement of cooking time.

Crispy Rhubarb Lemon Chicken Bake

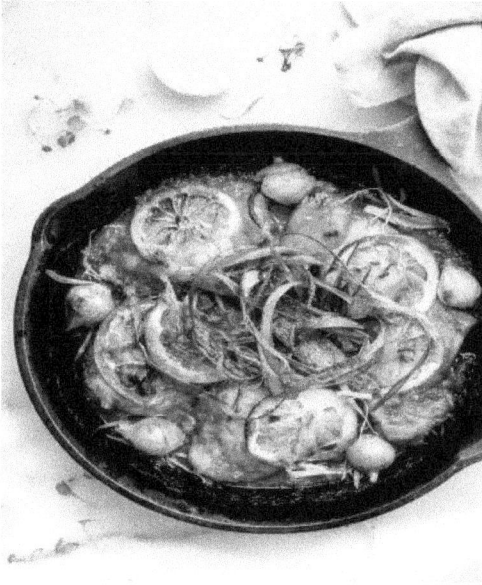

Ingredients:

1/4 c creamy balsamic dressing or vinaigrette

1/4 c tangy BBQ sauce

1/2 t salt

1/2 t pepper

1/4 c maple syrup

2 to 3 rhubarb stalks, shaved/peeled. Keep shavings for topping.

1 T lemon juice

2 garlic cloves

1.5 pounds skinless boneless chicken thighs, about 5 small thighs.

1 lemon

olive oil for pan fry

1 c pearled onions

Salt and Pepper to taste

Tarragon leaves or thyme to garnish

Optional 1/4 teaspoon garlic seasoning

Instructions:

1. Cooking temperature is 375 F.

2. Clean rhubarb stalks, trim ends, and use a vegetable peeler to peel off the red skin to create shavings. Set shavings aside for later.

3. Put the 2 to 3 small stalks in a blender with the BBQ sauce, dressing, syrup, and seasoning. Blend until creamy.

4. Clean and trim chicken thighs, then place somewhere else.

5. Put in the olive oil, 1 T of it, to oven safe or cast iron skillet.

6. Add in the rhubarb marinade and chicken thighs to the pan, squeeze fresh lemon juice on top.

7. Bring marinade to a quick bubble/boil. Once you see the edges start to caramelize on the pan, reduce or turn off heat.

8. Flip the chicken thighs over and place lemon slices on top of each thigh.

9. Add pearled onions to the pan and drizzle a little olive oil on top.

10. Add salt and pepper as desired.

11. 20 - 25 mins of cooking time.

12. While chicken is baking for the first 10 minutes, season the rhubarb shavings. Simply toss with a little oil, salt, pepper, and optional lemon pepper/lemon garlic.

13. Place rhubarb shavings on the greased baking sheet, and transfer to the oven when there are 15 minutes left of the chicken bake time. Toss shavings half way through to make sure they get crispy.

14. Once done cooking, place chicken thighs on a plate each. Add more marinade from the pan to the top of each chicken, then top with the crispy rhubarb shavings. Serve with the pearl onions.

15. Salt and pepper to taste.

16. Thyme to garnish!

Chapter 9: Tips to Reduce Inflammation

The biggest tip to reduce inflammation is changing the way you eat. We spoke about good foods to eat in Chapter 4, but here is a more in-depth look at some of the foods and other areas you can use to fight inflammation.

Turmeric: it almost seems like a fad; turmeric is "in" right now and causing a large movement for those who haven't heard of it. And for good reason! Turmeric contains a compound called "curcumin", which is specifically what gives this spice its anti-inflammatory powers. There is not much found in the ground spice, so it might be best to ask your doctor about taking supplements. However, its anti-inflammatory properties are still a good reason to use it liberally in different recipes. It tastes best with roasted veggies or even in smoothies and lattes!

Greens: leafy green vegetables have a high amount of magnesium, a mineral in which many people don't consume enough of. Low magnesium levels coincide with high inflammation, heart disease, and diabetes, so it's best to get a larger dose. And the best way to do that is to start eating more leafy greens!

Red/Blue/Purple: green isn't the only color that is good for you. There's a compound called anthocyanin, which is what gives produce its red, blue, and purple colors. Those that consume higher levels of this compound seem to have a lower measure of inflammatory activity. And it doesn't take much to achieve the necessary dose either! Just eating 1/3 cup of blackberries, 18 red grapes, or 1 cup of shredded red cabbage can provide about 40 mg of anthocyanins a day.

Nuts: nuts have a strong anti-inflammatory effect, due to their combination of antioxidants, fiber, and omega-3 fatty acids. Eating them regularly is best, usually, about 5 ounces spread out throughout the week.

Protein: eat protein at every meal! Most people eat a lot of protein during dinnertime but eating it for every meal throughout the day can help your liver detoxify all those bad chemicals that might be moving through your body. The best thing to do is focus on lean proteins, like fish, eggs, low fat dairy, chicken, and legumes.

Turn down the heat: interestingly enough, cooking meat at too high of a heat can form HCAs, or heterocyclic amines, and PAHs, or polycyclic aromatic hydrocarbons, which are inflammatory chemicals that can make your body more prone to getting cancer. So when cooking meat on the grill or stove, keep the temperature under 300 degrees Fahrenheit to help minimize these chemicals from forming.

There are also various things you can do besides eating healthily that will help to reduce inflammation:

Exercise: one of the biggest causes of inflammation is obesity. Getting more exercise and upping your activity is important to keep away inflammation; exercise improves lymphatic flow and circulation. You don't even have to actively be looking to lose weight, but simply be just active. This can include yard work, household chores, taking a walk, even parking in a spot that's further away from the store entrance can help. The most important part is to just get up and move. Focus on the enjoyment and not the calorie burn.

Get Rid of Stress: it's been shown that those who experience higher levels of stress tend to have more inflammation than those who don't. If you keep being stressed, then the constant damage to your heart rate and blood pressure causes inflammation. Those that take on stressful tasks in stride and learn how to deal with stress in a healthy way don't have to deal with high blood pressure and a higher heart rate. What can really help is taking some scheduled "me" time. You might not be able to control some things around you, but you can control how you spend your time. Making self-care a priority can actually go a long way towards easing your stress, which will in turn help with your inflammation.

Yoga: those that practice yoga regularly show levels of a lower rate of "interleukin-6" and "C-reactive protein". These are the two main markers of inflammation and typically aren't found in people that are new to yoga or don't practice regularly. By doing yoga about an hour and a half twice a week, you can prevent inflammation from happening. Yoga also reduces stress, which in turn also helps to reduce inflammation.

Get Enough Sleep: it's not exactly the lack of sleep, but how you behave when you're tired that causes inflammation. Not enough rest can make you more sensitive to stress, which in turn causes inflammation. It can make you feel quicker to anger, so you can change that mind set by either sleeping more or finding a more healthy conflict-resolution strategy.

Massage: massages are more than just a treat or something that high maintenance people do. A day at the spa might seem silly, but massages can actually help you to be healthy. They can lower the levels of two inflammation promoting hormones, decrease inflammatory substances, and lower stress hormones. It's possible to see results after just one massage, so it's definitely worth trying.

Green Tea: even if you're more of a coffee person, green tea has so many health benefits that it's worth trying. It's full of antioxidants that help reduce inflammation and inhibit stress. It might take a lot to actually see the results - maybe 4 to 6 cups daily - but even drinking one cup a day can help. Keep in mind that while green tea has a lot of antioxidants, it specifically targets inflammation that is caused by oxidation. So if that's not the reason for your inflammation, then green tea might not help reduce it.

Gadgets: a good night's sleep is important, and not having one can actually cause your inflammation to flare up. However, most people tend to be on their phones after they've gone to bed, which results in poor sleep. The light from your phone actually throws off your internal clock and makes it so much more difficult to actually be in a deep sleep. And sleeping badly can lead to an increase in inflammatory hormones, so try banning gadgets from the bedroom and see how it helps!

Sweet drinks: stay away from those sweetened drinks! It doesn't matter if the drink is diet, low calorie, regular, or sugar free; any beverage that has high fructose corn syrup and artificial sweeteners always lead to extremely high levels of insulin in the body. Higher insulin levels cause inflammation and other conditions like obesity and diabetes.

Filter water: drinking water is always the smart thing to do. It's important to stay hydrated; it helps keep you healthy, ups your metabolism, and even clears up your skin. However, sometimes tap water can contain chemicals that cause inflammation so filtering your water through a reverse osmosis water filter can help you to ensure that water is the only thing you're actually drinking.

Stay green: there are so many personal care products out there. From super cheap to extremely expensive, they all claim to be good for you and your body. But so many of them contain harsh chemicals that can contain inflammatory agents. And these chemicals can be found in not only in personal hygiene products but cleansers as well. The best thing to do is switch to phthalate-free products and lessen your exposure to possible inflammation.

Gratitude: practicing gratitude might seem like it doesn't have anything to do with inflammation or Rheumatoid Arthritis. However, it can help you to see your situation in a different light, which can, in turn, lessen stress and panic, and open you up to new solutions. Practicing gratitude changes your response to stress, which in turn helps to reduce inflammation markers. Gratitude makes people happier, improves their health, and helps to strengthen existing relationships.

Chapter 10: The Simple Guide to Anti-Inflammatory Supplements

While exercise, a different diet, stress management, and good sleep can all help reduce inflammation, sometimes you need a little something extra. And that's where supplements come in. They can be very useful and provide additional support. It's important to remember that if you want to try supplements, then you should purchase them from a manufacturer with a good reputation and follow the correct dosage instructions. You should also first check with your doctor because there could be negative side effects if you already take meds or if you have a pre-existing condition. There are a few different kinds that can help:

Curcumin: Found in turmeric, curcumin has many impressive benefits. It has the ability to lower inflammation found in many conditions, specifically those with Rheumatoid Arthritis and Osteoarthritis. There have actually been studies done on those who have a metabolic syndrome. They consumed curcumin and had a surprising amount of reduced levels of inflammation, compared to others who only received a placebo in place of the curcumin. Another study had a large number of people that had tumors suspected of being cancerous take 150 mg, and it showed that their quality of life increased and their inflammatory levels decreased. Curcumin happens to not absorb well when it's taken on its own but taking it with a compound called piperine can increase curcumin's absorption by about 2,000 percent. Some of the supplements have bioperine, and it works in a similar way to piperine. So by looking for a supplement that has both curcumin and bioperine, you'll be able to make sure you're ingesting enough curcumin to make a difference for your inflammation.

The recommended dosage of curcumin is 100 to 500 mg taken daily when taken with piperine or bioperine. It's possible to take at most 10 grams daily and still be considered a safe amount but doing so has the possibility of causing side effects in the digestive area. Curcumin isn't recommended for pregnant women.

Alpha-Lipoic Acid: Alpha-lipoic acid has an important job in your body's production of energy and metabolism. It can also double its function by being an antioxidant, and protects from damage within the body's cells, and helps to increase the levels from more antioxidants, like vitamin E and vitamin C. Reducing inflammation linked to insulin resistance, liver and heart disease, and many other conditions, this supplement has some great health benefits. It even helps lower several different markers of inflammation and their blood levels, including ICAM-1 and IL-6. It's really good to take for those suffering specifically with heart disease.

The recommended dosage is 300 to 600 mg daily. Taking it at the recommended dosage doesn't cause any side effects, and it's possible to take the full amount of 600 mg daily with no issues. Be on the lookout and monitor your blood sugar levels if you also take diabetes medications. Alpha-lipoic acid is best if taken when not pregnant.

Fish Oil: these supplements are fantastic and extremely helpful. They have what's called "omega-3 fatty acids", and these are specifically important for keeping you in your best health. Fish oil supplements have the ability to reduce inflammation that is found within diabetes, and several more disorders. There are two versions of omega-3s that can be especially beneficial. There is what's called eicosatetraenoic acid, or EPA, and docosahexaenoic acid, or DHA. DHA is specifically beneficial because it has effects that decrease cytokine levels, ensures a healthy gut, and is anti-inflammatory. Also, it's very helpful after exercising; it can reduce inflammation and muscle damage due to strenuous activity.

The recommended dosage of fish oil supplements is 1 to 1.5 grams. The best thing to do is look for supplements with undetectable mercury content. Mercury isn't bad to digest, per se, but too much of it can be harmful. Be careful, because it's possible to cause blood thinning when taking fish oil. Because of this, fish oil supplements aren't recommended when you're taking aspirin or any other blood thinners. The only exception is if a doctor has already authorized it.

Ginger: ginger is incredible and has so many health benefits. It's most commonly ground into a powder as a spice and added to recipes for extra flavor. However, ginger does more than just taste great! It's commonly used to treat nausea and indigestion. It's fantastic for morning sickness, motion sickness, and any stomach issues. That's why many people drink Ginger Ale when sick; the ginger in the soda really does help them to feel better. Two components found in ginger are zingerone and gingerol, which can decrease inflammation that is linked to kidney damage, diabetes, breast cancer, and colitis. When those that have diabetes took 1,600 mg of ginger every day, they found that their problematic levels significantly decreased. In a different study, it was discovered that when women that have breast cancer ingested supplements with ginger, they ended up with lower levels of IL-6 and CRP. It was especially beneficial when combining the supplements with exercising. In fact, ginger is so helpful that it can even decrease muscle soreness and inflammation after exercise.

The recommended dosage is taking 1 gram every day. It's fine if you end up taking 2 grams instead. Consuming ginger in higher doses, however, can possibly cause your blood to thin. Therefore, if you're taking any blood thinners, like aspirin, then ginger supplements probably aren't in your best interest, unless your doctor has said it's fine.

Resveratrol: this antioxidant is found within blueberries, grapes, and any other purple-skinned type of fruit. It's not just found in fruit with purple skin, however! Although these two might seem like they have nothing to do with each other, you can also find resveratrol in red wine and peanuts! These supplements can help to lower swelling and inflammation that those with insulin resistance have. One study done gave 500 mg of resveratrol daily to people who have ulcerative colitis. They saw a decrease in their inflammation markers TNF, CRP, and NF-kB and their overall symptoms improved. Another study gave resveratrol supplements to people with obesity and saw their inflammatory markers, blood sugar, and triglycerides significantly lowered. Many people believe that drinking a glass of red wine every day is healthy. And while the resveratrol found in red wine has health benefits, the amount really isn't high enough to make a difference. Red wine actually has no more 13 mg in every liter or 34 ounces. One bottle of red wine is about 25 ounces, so there is less than 13 mg of resveratrol in one bottle of wine. The health benefits found in resveratrol typically happen when people consume at least 150 mg. Basically, in order to get the right amount of resveratrol, you would need to drink about 3 gallons of wine, or around 13 bottles, daily. Definitely not a good recommendation!

The right dose of resveratrol is 150 to 500 mg per day. There are no possible negative effects when taking the right dose. However, it's possible to have digestive issues when ingesting larger amounts, about 5 grams every day. Resveratrol supplements aren't recommended for those taking blood thinning medications unless they have approval from their doctor.

Spirulina: Interestingly, spirulina is actually an algae, typically a blue-green color. It's an antioxidant, and has anti-inflammatory properties, strengthens the immune system, and leads to healthier aging. Studies done have shown taking spirulina can improve inflammatory marker, immune function, and anemia. Those that have diabetes took 8 grams of spirulina daily for 12 weeks, and the results were very positive. Their inflammation levels were actually reduced, and they saw an increase in the levels of their adiponectin (a hormone that levels out fat metabolism and blood sugar). Basically, taking spirulina is good!

The recommended dose of spirulina is 1 to 8 grams per day. Besides allergy reactions, there are no potential side effects when taking the recommended dosage. Spirulina isn't recommended for those with allergies to spirulina or algae and those with immune system disorders.

Berberine: taken from several anti-diabetic plants, including the plant Berberis Aristate, berberine is most well-known today for being a potent AMPK inducer. It works similar to the medicine Metformin and other similar pharmaceutical medicines, and also is also known throughout history as being called an herbal Imodium. Basically, it's similar to a pharmaceutical anti-diarrhea drug. It has the ability to decrease inflammatory responses which tend to happen the most frequently in a person's intestines. In addition to helping with diarrhea and intestinal bacteria, studies have also shown berberine can help to alleviate ulcerative colitis. Those who are suffering from irritable bowel syndrome, or IBS, can take berberine supplements to help reduce diarrhea and other symptoms. This is because both irritable bowel syndrome and ulcerative colitis are inflammatory conditions that are found in the intestines. Berberine not only helps tremendously with intestinal inflammation but also with whole body anti-inflammatory properties and benefits blood glucose management. Which makes berberine a pretty special anti-inflammatory!

Quercetin: this supplement is a good choice if you have chronic inflammation and a history of taking NSAIDs. Quercetin has a sort of protective effect on the liver, which is good because NSAID causes negative issues within that organ. Quercetin can be found in foods like apples, berries, and some teas, and in supplement form. It protects brain neurons from degeneration which can lead to cognitive diseases like dementia and also has an anti-cancer effect.

Chondroitin: a component of human connective tissue, chondroitin is supplemented with a form derived from certain animals. It has pain decreasing effects on the body and reduces inflammation. Combining it with glucosamine allows chondroitin to be the most effective and helps to reduce pain in people who suffer from arthritis. A study was done where people with joint pain took a combination of chondroitin and glucosamine for a total of 3 months. Amazingly, NSAID use was decreased by 37 percent, which happened to coincide with a reduction in pain.

MSM: an organic and sulfuric compound found in every cell of the body, MSM has anti-inflammatory and pain reducing effects. It's best when working simultaneously with glucosamine and chondroitin, and works in the body's nerve tissue, skin, and joints. It can actually be used for metabolic disease and obesity; studies have shown it leads to lower inflammation associated with obesity, better blood sugar management, and an increased sensitivity to insulin.

Boswellia: a plant extract that has incredible anti-inflammatory effects in the body, Boswellia has been shown that it decreases the sensation of pain in healthy people, plus those with chronic pain due to joint issues like arthritis. A big thing to note and remember is that Boswellia has a protective effect on the liver and gut, which helps to lower oxidative stress. It's even been thought to be protective against cancer and can help to reduce symptoms of every and all inflammatory condition. A study was done where those with osteoarthritis took Boswellia had a decrease of pain and symptoms of osteoarthritis, which helped them to live a better quality of life and achieve higher physical activity.

Unfortunately, there are several supplements which aren't able to help inflammation and can, in fact, make it worse. Technically any supplement can be an anti-inflammatory; inflammation is a very large process and many things can happen in the body that can be called "inflammation". Even Ibuprofen can be considered an anti-inflammatory. Specific supplements that are marketed towards being anti-inflammatory can really just be hyped up for the benefits that they could maybe give. It's better to use supplements that you know for sure will work. These supplements, while not bad for you, probably won't make things better:

Green Tea: green tea, and catechins in general, have no real potency in regards to being able to reduce inflammation. Catechin is a term that is used to refer to molecules that look very similar to each other. They are commonly found either in dark chocolate with epicatechin, or in green tea with epigallocatechin-gallate. These specific two molecules, and in general catechins themselves, are strong antioxidants with great benefits to the body's blood flow. However, there is a difference between anti-inflammatory and antioxidant, but at some point, people started to assume that they were similar enough to call them both supplements to help inflammation. There are a few instances of inflammation that has been caused by oxidation, which is why an antioxidant can help. Because of this, most people have started to assume that green tea, being an antioxidant, will help with all forms of inflammation. It's important to know exactly what you have that is causing inflammation, and whether the green tea will actually help or not.

Acai/exotic sounding fruit: fruits and vegetables are always good to eat. Most don't like eating vegetables though and get tired of eating the same boring fruit over and over again. So why not try something interesting and exotic? The problem with that is these exotic fruits have no indication of actually helping inflammation. They might be really tasty and could possibly have health benefits, but nothing specific has been tested. The best thing to do is just eat some vegetables that have anti-inflammatory properties and eat the exotic fruit for taste.

Chaparral: some supplements are specifically bad for your liver, which include Kombucha tea, arnica, and chaparral. In fact, chaparral can cause liver toxicity, especially when combined with methotrexate, which is a commonly prescribed drug that can cause liver damage with its side effects.

Thunder god vine: this supplement can specifically ease your Rheumatoid Arthritis symptoms, but it causes a lot of side effects so many would consider it not worth the risk. You would have to deal with diarrhea, severe nausea, and respiratory infections, so the cons definitely outweigh the pros.

Chapter 11: Building Your Anti-Inflammatory Lifestyle

We've already talked about the importance of eating right, exercising, and stress relief. But maybe you're not quite sure how to get started. It can all seem overwhelming and like there's just too much information thrown at you. So here's a breakdown with some tips and ideas on how to get started with the Anti-Inflammatory Lifestyle!

Eat healthily:

Lots of fruits and vegetables

Eat the better for you meats, which are the leaner proteins

Don't eat all those processed food/ refined sugars

Add some spice to your meals

Exercise:

Take a walk

Try a new sport

Go for a bike ride

Join a yoga class or try at home

Join your local recreation center

Creative outlets:

Join an art club

Pick up your camera and start photographing

Try a DIY project at home

Doodle

Visit a museum, craft show, or farmer's market

Practice Positivity:

Write down positive thoughts in a journal every day

Practice gratitude

Compliment a stranger

Compliment yourself. This one might seem silly, but we are our own worst enemies, and sometimes you need a reminder that you're worth it.

Focus on the good by denying yourself the right to complain about things.

Conclusion

The next step is to make a plan! Put together a meal plan for the week that includes all the foods spoken about in this book. By making an actual menu for the week, you'll be less likely to eat foods that are bad for you and that will cause inflammation. Stick with foods that help reduce your pain and stay away from foods you know will cause it. Start an elimination diet and really pinpoint which foods actually hurt you and your body.

And not only should you plan your meals for the week, but also figure out a plan for your stress and exercises you can do to counter it. Journaling will help you to stay on track, and you can write down your goals for each week. Go on a walk every morning/evening, weed your garden, do yoga; whatever you decide, make sure it's something you actually like and will stick with. It can be difficult to start a new habit, no matter how much you know it will help your health to improve. But the important thing is to keep up with it, and soon you'll be eating healthy and actually be able to see improvements!

Remember, you're stronger than you think and a bad day doesn't equal a bad life!

Finally, if you found this book useful in any way, a review on Amazon is always appreciated!

www.ingramcontent.com/pod-product-compliance
Lightning Source LLC
Chambersburg PA
CBHW050723030426
42336CB00012B/1397